My Baby Hijacked My Body, Now I Want It Back!

Michelle Ishio
BA, CPT, CAFS

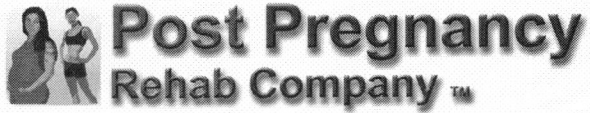 **Post Pregnancy**
Rehab Company ™

PostPregnancyRehab.com

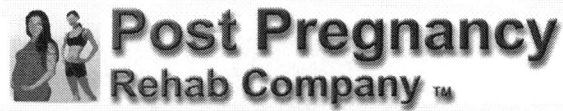

Post Pregnancy Rehab Company
Rehab   Fitness   Wellness

www.PostPregnancyRehab.com

Published by MKI World Wide Publishing   *(division of MKI World Wide)*

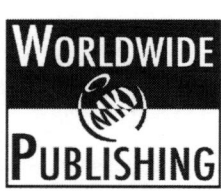   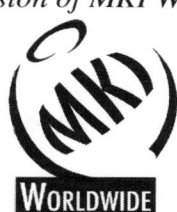

Book Cover/Graphic Design Credit: Michelle Ishio
Cover and Interior Photography Credit: Vincent Calloway

ISBN: 978-0991440528

Printed in the U.S.A.

Table of Contents

<u>Golden Rule for Moms</u>

"I AM as IMPORTANT as my children".
Do for ourselves as we do for our children.
It doesn't have to equal the same amount of time,
but it has to equal the same amount of care.

Awareness that you have the ability and responsibility to design the ambiance of your life is powerful wisdom to have; its creativity and productivity are endless.

Dedication

This book is dedicated to my children Kiyomi, Emiko, and Miya.

Having Kiyomi gave me the inspiration to vision and create the
Ishio Method ™ – Post Pregnancy Rehab Principles and Protocols,
the Sillo Belly Wrap ™, and PostPregnancyRehab.com.
Emi and Miya confirmed its necessity, and effectiveness ☺.

Introduction

Welcome to one of the most significant milestones of your life…becoming a mother!

I congratulate you for taking the initiative with taking care of yourself, your body, and your recovery. Understanding the importance of self-care, and that "you matter too", is an extremely positive step necessary towards recovering properly.

Great news is that by understanding and applying the Ishio Method – Post Pregnancy Rehab Key Principles and Protocols TM, not only can you return to your pre-pregnancy state, but you can also improve from before you ever had a baby.

I know that the term "post pregnancy rehab" is a new term that's not really used, but I do call it "post pregnancy rehab" with full conviction. My perspectives and concepts comes from my personal experience of having 3 little ones myself, as well, 2 decades as a professional in the fitness and wellness field specializing in women's health, and even longer than that, as an elite level multi-sport athlete.

When athletes get injured with common sports specific injuries, we have an immediate protocol system put in place on what to do to lessen the severity of the injury, and also have the speediest recoveries. We make it a priority to nurture ourselves so we can get back to functioning at optimum levels once again. There are also mandatory rehab protocols put in place for countless medical procedures. I playfully call pregnancy and delivery an "injury in slow motion", and know that post-pregnancy mothers vitally need rehab structured type of care available also.

When I was pregnant and had my first child, I couldn't believe how yucky, and for how long, my body felt. I'm not talking simply about body fat, or a "puffy" belly either; I'm talking about all the hidden stuff that happens with our muscle functions, body aches, abrupt changes in hormones, (i.e. sleep disturbances, postpartum depression), posture, etc. Just because our body, naturally, without conscious effort, changes for the miracles of pregnancy and delivery, that doesn't mean that it will naturally, without conscious effort, go back to the way it was before either; we need to purposefully help our bodies recover and prosper, or else it won't.

As with athletes and general post-operative patients, mothers need a specific rehab protocol system, and clear wellness options, in place ahead of time. Many of us have to stop simply "getting by", or "hoping what we are doing is working", or "barely surviving"; which all of this only gets harder with each new baby we have.

This is exactly why I started PostPregnancyRehab.com, created the Ishio Method TM – Post Pregnancy Rehab Key Principles and Protocols TM, and wrote *My Baby Hijacked My Body, Now I Want It Back!* My purpose is to help improve mother's lives; by offering clear and simple information, removing some confusion and doubts, and offering solutions for post pregnancy physical rehab, and wellness necessities.

Even if a few years has gone by since your child was born, don't worry, it is never too late to benefit from this recovery program; you WILL still achieve considerable positive improvements.

Please Note: You will see some repeated information in this book; this is not by accident. They are intentionally repeated because I want to stress certain important facts, and concepts.

Visit www.PostPregnancyRehab.com for additional FREE support.

For those that "graduate" from the Ishio Method – Post Pregnancy Rehab Program, you have the option of continued support through our Michelle Ishio Fit Club at MichelleIshio.com.

<u>Golden Rule for Moms</u>

"I AM as IMPORTANT as my children".
Do for ourselves as we do for our children.
It doesn't have to equal the same amount of time,
but it has to equal the same amount of care.

Awareness that you have the ability and responsibility to design the ambiance of your life is powerful wisdom to have; its creativity and productivity are endless.

Section One - Pregnancy

Chapter One:

Things To Consider During Pregnancy To Help With Recovery

Healthy Weight Gain

Now-a-days, the common recommended weight gain for "healthy weight" individuals is 25 - 35lbs. Ultimately, the "optimal weight" gain differs from mother to mother depending on her weight/health at the time of pregnancy, so consulting your doctor as to what's best for your personal case is the best direction to go.

The first pro-active thing you can do for your "Post-Pregnancy Rehab" is to start while you are pregnant, and not gain the unnecessary extra pounds/fat that your pregnancy doesn't require.

Caloric Needs Of Pregnancy

"Eating for two"

I don't want to take the fun out of this saying, but contrary to this saying, you are NOT eating for two.

The only extra caloric requirement to maintain a healthy pregnancy is an extra 300 calories per day. This extra requirement isn't even really necessary until you are in your 2nd and 3rd trimesters.

So why do many of us have the hormonal shifts that make us want to eat like we are literally eating for two? The answer is "just because"…what a mean trick isn't it?!

An example for the 300 calories:

* A scoop of regular ice cream and a medium size piece of fruit.
* A plain bagel with thin cream cheese.
* A serving of yogurt and piece of cheese.

Now that you see how little "extra" food the 300 calories really is, can you see how it is easy for so many Moms to exceed the "weight gain" necessary for pregnancy?

1

Exercise

Continue exercising, with necessary modifications for your different stages of pregnancy. If you are not currently exercising, you may want to include a mild stretching, walking, and strength training routine, to have your body in better physical balance during a time when it is rapidly changing. Ultimately, what exercises you can continue or start doing all depends on your health, what you were doing before pregnancy, and also what type of pregnancy you are having. Consult with you doctor.

Exercise can help with your self-assurance during a time when your body is rapidly changing, help alleviate body aches, reduce unhealthy cravings, lessen muscle loss, and provide confidence for your pregnancy, delivery, and recovery.

Pregnancy Exercise Standard Guidelines
ACOG Guidelines 2002 (American College of Obstetricians and Gynecologists)

1. During pregnancy, women can continue to exercise. It is noted that there are health benefits with mild to moderate exercise. Participating in some form of exercise regularly is recommended.

2. Women should avoid exercise in the supine position after the 1st trimester. Supine position is when you are laying down on your back. This position is associated with decreased blood flow to the uterus/baby.

3. Long periods of motionless standing should be avoided.

4. Pregnant women should not exercise until exhaustion. Please be aware of the decreased oxygen available for aerobic exercise during pregnancy.

5. Any type of exercise involving potential to lose balance and falling, or any type of abdominal trauma should be avoided.

6. Women who exercise during pregnancy should be particularly careful in getting enough calories and nutrition in their daily diet.

7. When exercising, it is important to offset the extra heat by making sure you stay well hydrated and wear appropriate clothing. This is especially important during the first trimester.

8. Many of the physical pregnancy traits continue for weeks postpartum, so pre-pregnancy exercise routines should be resumed gradually based on each individual woman's physical abilities.

Avoid these movements while exercising:

1. Compromising joint movements. Your joints are looser, and you can more easily injury your joints even if the movements are the same as before you were pregnant.

2. High impact movements. Your baby's environment is critical, so you don't want to potentially rupture the amniotic sac.

3. Twisting and rapid direction change. Same reason as #1 and #2.

4. Exercise that requires fine balance. Postural changes, looser joints, etc, will shift throughout the pregnancy, causing balance to shift as well.

5. Exercises that require too much abdominal strength. You don't want to aggravate the abdominal separation that is already being created with the growing belly. Depending on the exertion/weight applied, you can potentially permanently "rip" your abdominal muscles from the fascia skin, causing it to never fully go back to the position it started out at before pregnancy.

Don't participate in exercise if any of these apply:

* Significant heart disease
* Restrictive lung disease
* Incompetent cervix
* Carrying multiple babies at risk for premature labor
* Recurrent second or third trimester bleeding
* Placenta previa after 26 weeks of pregnancy
* Premature labor during current pregnancy
* Ruptured membranes
* Preeclampsia/pregnancy induced hypertension

Warning signs to stop exercising while pregnant:

* Vaginal bleeding
* Shortness of breath prior to exertion
* Dizziness
* Headache
* Chest pain
* Muscle weakness
* Calf pain or swelling (need to rule out swelling of vein due to a blood clot)
* Preterm labor
* Decreased fetal movement
* Amniotic fluid leakage

Pelvic Floor Muscle Health

Read and apply Chapters 2, 3, and 4.

By getting early familiarity, and applying the Ishio Method - Key Principles and Pelvic Floor Exercise Protocol ᴛᴍ before delivery, you can get a head start with gaining great habits, and the body awareness necessary for a smoother post pregnancy recovery; you will only have to "reacquaint" yourself with what you need to do, rather than learning something "brand new" while caring for a new baby.

At the very least, learn and start applying Ishio Method ™ – Post-Pregnancy Rehab Principles #1, #2, and #3. These 3 principles alone will have you well on your way with your abdominal and pelvic floor recovery after delivering your baby; you can apply these principles no matter where, or what you are doing.

Breast Care During Pregnancy

Wear supportive garments, (bras), <u>at all times</u>, day and night.

<u>While sleeping</u>: wear a bra since the density of your breasts will increase in weight, which will increase the pulling/stretching on the tissues and ligaments at all times.

<u>While exercising</u>: wear a bra underneath a jog bra since you want extra support. It doesn't matter even if your have smaller sized breasts, bouncing is bouncing, and stretching is stretching. Your breasts already have to "stretch" while growing to accommodate breastfeeding, and the last thing you want is additional unnecessary stretching from exercising.

For other important breast care information after pregnancy, refer to **Chapter 7 – Skin Care – Breast care.**

Skin Care During Pregnancy (stretch marks, face malasma)

<u>Stretch Marks:</u>

* In order to help prevent, or lessen the severity of stretch marks, it is important not gain more weight then the recommended 25-35 lbs.

* Another recommendation for stretch marks is, you want to avoid any unnecessary rapid weight gain in a short period of time, (first and second trimester). In the last trimester, you will already have the most and fastest weight/size gain due to the fact that this is when the baby's bones/size are growing most rapidly. Keeping your weight gain appropriately gradual up until the last few months will help.

* Support you skin's growth with proper nutrition and hydration throughout your pregnancy.

Even if a woman follows good preventative measures for stretch marks, some women may still get stretch marks because it's part of their DNA susceptibility; the good news is that by following preventative measures, you will definitely lessen its severity. Just the same, just because your Mother has stretch marks doesn't automatically mean you will too, because maybe your Mother wasn't properly following preventative measures herself.

Face Malasma (pregnancy mask):

"Pregnancy mask" is brown pigmentation on your face. You can look up images of "pregnancy face malasma" on the internet to see what this looks like.

During pregnancy, your body produces extra amounts of melanin, which cause hyper pigmentation, (extra browning in various areas of your skin). Melanin is the chemical that protects your skin, and gives you that "tan" color when your body is exposed to the sun. Common spots for pregnancy mask are under the eyes, cheekbones, and above the lip, although it can happen anywhere, such as the forehead.

To help lessen the effects of pregnancy mask, wear sunscreen daily, SPF 30 is recommended. Re-apply if continually staying outdoors or direct sunlight is coming through your windows, (i.e. car, office, etc).

The most effective way to help lessen the effects of pregnancy mask, (along with sunscreen), is to provide yourself shade by wearing a hat under direct sunlight.

For other important skin information, refer to **Chapter 7 – Skin Care – Stretch Marks and Malasma.**

Upper back, Lower back, Leg, Feet – Posture and/or Pain

To help alleviate any upper back, lower back, leg, or feet pain, refer to **Chapter 6 - Balansu Therapy TM**, for any postural corrections and/or stretches available for you to do.

Note: please consult with a physician to make sure you are in good physical health to try any of the stretches/postural corrections contained in this program. As well, do not do any strength exercises that would compromise your pregnancy, nor do any exercise that has you laying down on your back after your 1ˢᵗ trimester, (i.e. laying down on your back and elevating you legs for leg pain relief; instead you will elevate your legs while seated).

<u>Golden Rule for Moms</u>

"I AM as IMPORTANT as my children".
Do for ourselves as we do for our children.
It doesn't have to equal the same amount of time,
but it has to equal the same amount of care.

Awareness that you have the ability and responsibility to design the ambiance of your life is powerful wisdom to have; its creativity and productivity are endless.

Section Two - Post-Pregnancy

Chapter Two:

Ishio Method – Post Pregnancy Rehab Key Principles ™

Key Principles:

Principle #1: Core Posture ™
Principle #2: Surge Posture ™
Principle #3: Set Posture ™
Principle #4: Breath Posture ™

But first, so the Key Principles will make easier sense…

Did You Know That Our Pelvic Floor Muscles Are Part Of Our Core?

Our "Core System" in a Nutshell: let's look at our "core system" as being a rectangle in the middle of our gut.

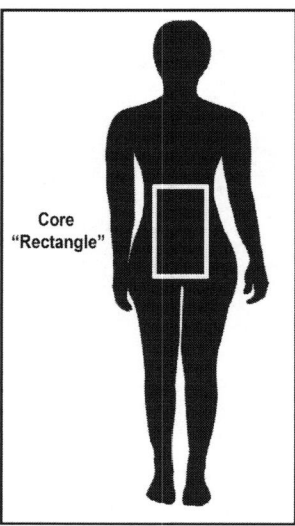

Our pelvic floor muscles are the "bottom" of our "core rectangle", (the muscles that surround or are, our urethra, anus, and vagina).

Our diaphragm is the "top" of our "core rectangle", (main muscle that helps us with breathing).

Our abdominal muscles are the "front and sides" of our "core rectangle", (our "6-pack", and the muscles that wrap around the sides of our waist).

Our back muscles are the "back" of our "core rectangle", (the muscles that surround our spine).

This All Matters Because Why?

Pelvic floor and abdominal muscles are not muscles that stand alone working by itself, it affects and is affected by the other muscles just mentioned in the "core rectangle"; determining how effectively the groups of muscles works individually, and with each other.

This means that for thorough post pregnancy pelvic floor and abdominal muscles rehabbing, we need to work all groups in our "core rectangle" together, at the same time. Don't worry, it's not as tricky as it sounds; basically, this can be done if you follow the Ishio Method – Post-Pregnancy Rehab Principles ™.

When your "core rectangle" is properly interacting with each other, this will allow you to be "exercising" your abs and pelvic floor muscles even while simply moving through normal daily movements. Then of course when formally exercising, this mid-section posture will benefit you with even better impact.

For FYI: everything that was just described above about our "core rectangle" is our "pelvic core neuromuscular system". Don't worry though, as promised, I will deliver simplified information on what needs to be done. **The Ishio Method – Post Pregnancy Rehab Key Principles ™ ARE what helps you use your "pelvic core neuromuscular system" more effectively, which greatly helps you properly rehab your post pregnancy abs and pelvic floor muscles.**

Why Is It Critical To Rehab The Pelvic Floor Muscles?

Besides properly contributing to the functioning of the entire "core system"…

To Help Heal Tears: By doing pelvic floor exercises, we bring blood flow, (and it's healing properties), to the torn muscles, speeding up healing; light movements such as those from pelvic floor exercises, also speeds up our body's physical healing mechanisms. When we have skin or muscle tears from delivering our baby, often times, our doctors stich up those tears; but we also can have muscle tears that are internal, (not visibly seen because our skin isn't torn). These torn muscles can only heal as "closed up" as possible, by doing consistent pelvic floor exercises, and allowing our muscles to get back as much of it's pre-delivery muscle integrity as it can, so the tears can heal as close to each other as possible.

Prevent Urinary Incontinence: When you hear a woman complain about having "an accidental leak" when she sneezed, that is one of the signs of having weak pelvic floor muscles. This is not something that we have to accept as a permanent condition because we had babies, and this can be prevented or corrected.

I would like to also note that urinary incontinence doesn't only happen because the muscles are now weaker in the pelvis floor area, but it's also because Mom's need to "re-train" their pelvic floor muscle's reaction to exertion; more on "muscle reaction" will be explained later in this chapter.

Prevent Organ Prolapse: Connective tissues, (i.e. ligaments), hold up the organs in our body. Our pelvis floor muscles also helps prop up some of our organs, (i.e. uterus and bladder). Carrying a growing baby pushes our organs upwards/downwards, as well, carrying and delivering a baby stretches the connective tissues holding our organs in place, and stretches our muscles too.

After delivery, we have gravity against us in the sense that everything is being "pulled downwards", and our organs, (with stretched out connective tissues), are lying on top of our now weak vaginal wall. By doing the rehab exercises to help re-strengthen the pelvic floor muscles, it will help "prop" these organs up.

<u>Symptoms</u> that you can look for to tell you if you may be suffering from organ prolapse are: feeling of pelvic fullness or pressure, incontinence, discomfort with intercourse, pain or bleeding from the vagina that is not menses related, lower back pain, and/or constipation. See your OBGYN for confirmation.

<u>Maintain a Healthy Sex Life</u>: If there is moderate to significant looseness in the vagina, there will be significant enough decrease in stimulation for both the man and the woman. As with urinary incontinence, this is not something that we have to accept as a permanent condition because we had babies, this can be corrected.

When a woman has control of her pelvic floor muscles, (and specifically the vaginal muscle), she can draw better blood flow to the area, control the stimulation that she feels, and have more confidence and awareness with her own body; all of which promotes a better over-all experience and orgasms. Although sex is not "everything" for a healthy relationship, it is an important part.

Why Is It Critical To Rehab The Abdominal Muscles?

Besides properly contributing to the functioning of the entire "core system"…

<u>Prevent back pain</u>: Every movement we make requires core movement. Without strong abdominal muscles, our back has to make up for what are abdominals are not contributing towards our core stability, which is often times why we end up with chronic back pain.

<u>To get our "armor" back</u>: Our abdominal muscles protect our organs, and when they are strong, we have good protection. If we have a large enough gap between our 6-pack halves, (diastasis recti), we have a weak spot that not doesn't properly protect our organs. We also have a very high risk of having or eventually getting a hernia, (internal tissues protruding).

<u>For Balance/Strength</u>: Every movement we make requires core movement. When the back and/or abdominal muscles are weak, then our over-all balance and strength with all movements are compromised.

<u>For Physique</u>: Even if we were to decrease our body fat to a healthy level, if we do not rehab our abdominal muscles properly, then our belly will still protrude as if we were still pregnant. Often enough, I have clients come to me and say, "I still look pregnant even after a year since I had my baby, how do I get rid of this belly fat?" Many times, the excess protruding belly is in fact the abdominal muscle protruding, not just body fat. Any excess body fat on top of the protruding abdominal muscles just gives the illusion of the fat being the culprit for that "still pregnant" look, when in reality it is also "un-rehabbed" muscle.

Important Note: In some cases, the protruding belly is also because a Mom may be suffering from a moderate to severe case of diastasis recti. Diastasis recti is a condition that usually doesn't cause pain, and where both halves of the "six-pack" do not come back together properly. In severe cases, it's highly recommended that a Mom get surgery to bring the two halves together, so as not to cause other complications in the future.

Note: All the issues just noted on the previous page are not just issues that affect new mothers; many women, (who have never even had children), also can suffer from them. As we age, the muscles all over our body will weaken unless we regularly strength exercise them, (which also includes our pelvic floor and abdominal muscles).

A Tad More About The Pelvic Floor Muscles

Sometimes the pelvic floor muscles are described as a "basket" that holds our bottom area together and up. Our pelvic floor muscles also travels up, (around our rectum, vaginal wall, urethra), within this "basket" as well.

Below is a model of the pelvic floor muscles attached to a pelvis bone. Notice that if the model was to "stand up", how the muscles are like a "basket".

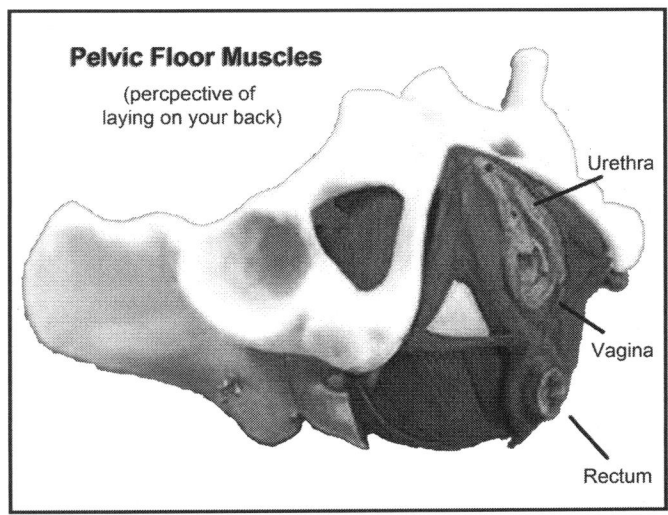

Pelvic Floor Muscles
(percpective of laying on your back)

Urethra

Vagina

Rectum

Below is a quick illustration of the pelvic floor muscles. The shaded areas are the muscles, and notice how it goes "upwards" in our body.

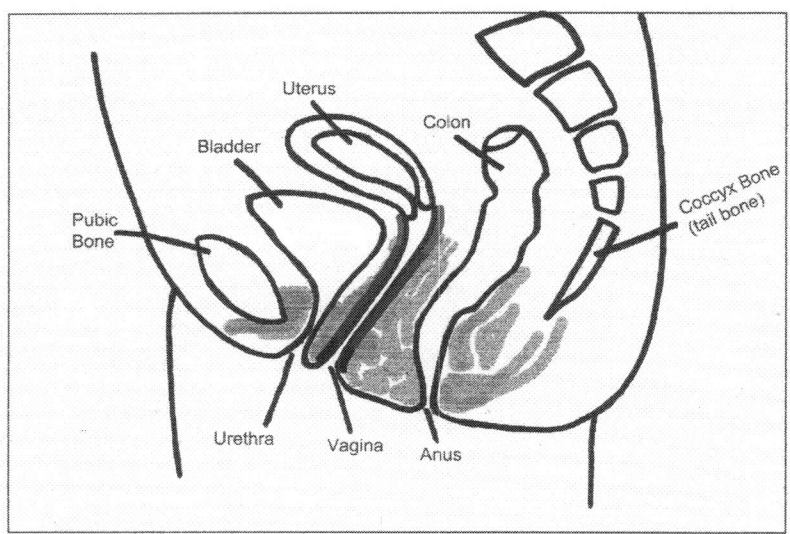

About "Kegels"

Dr. Arnold Kegel introduced the "Kegels". Kegels are the basic and conscious tightening of the pelvis floor muscles, first published in 1948. When doing "Kegels", you are contracting the many groups of muscles in the pelvic floor muscles "basket".

The basic explanation that's being used now-a-days to explain how to do "Kegels" are, when urinating, try to stop the flow of urine during midstream. Since it's been noted that it's not a good idea to regularly "stop the flow of urine midstream" because in the long run it weakens your pelvic floor muscles, my suggestion is to use the bathroom as you normally would, and at the very end when your bladder is nearly empty, THEN "stop the flow of urine"; this way, you won't be applying unnecessary pressure on your pelvic floor muscles. The muscles you are using to stop urinating are part of your pelvic floor muscles.

The popular suggestions for "Kegels" that have been circulating out there for new Moms are roughly like this: "squeeze your pelvic floor muscles and hold for a count of 5 seconds, then relax, then repeat 5 - 10 times; eventually you want to be able to squeeze for 10 seconds at a time."

The "popular Kegels" is a great introduction to becoming familiar with your pelvic floor muscles if you were not familiar before, and it's better than doing nothing, but for true recovery after having been stretched out carrying and delivering a baby, we need a more thorough "rehab protocol" if we are to realistically get back to our pre-pregnancy state.

Why We <u>Need</u> To Do <u>More</u> Than Just "Kegels"

1. Our pelvic floor muscles don't stand alone on it's own; the muscles are attached to bone, tissue, and other muscles, so we need to consider what/where it is attached to. Through studies, we know that our pelvic floor muscles can contract more efficiently when in certain positions, which is why understanding Core Posture TM, (Ishio Method – Key Principle #1), makes a major difference.

2. After our muscles has been pressured for months, and stretched out dramatically, we need to re-calibrate our muscle's reaction to exertion. We need to make sure we aren't subconsciously reinforcing "stretching out/open" muscle movements during normal day-to-day movements, and especially during exercise. Doing "Kegels" randomly does not teach our mind-body to re-calibrate our muscle's reactions, which is why understanding and doing Surge Postures TM, (Ishio Method Principle #2), is necessary.

3. As with the concept of number 2 above, since our muscles have been pressured and stretched out dramatically, we need to re-calibrate our body as to where those muscles are supposed to "sit" within our body when we are "at rest". (Set Posture TM – Ishio Method Principle #3)

4. Breathing properly helps pretty much everything, (speaking, exercising, stress management, better memory, etc), and it is now known that breathing properly also matters with how effectively we engage our pelvic floor muscles. Because our diaphragm is the "top part" of our "core rectangle", when one side is not efficient, it affects the efficiency of its other sides. (Breath Posture TM - Ishio Method Principle #4)

5. We need to have a specific rehab protocol that we start applying soon after delivery, just as post-operation patients do after surgery. We should seize the time when our body's hormones are dramatically helping with the recovery process. Having limited information on what we can do for ourselves, that we apply randomly, is not sufficient for what our body just went through; we need a more precise plan that we can use to target our specific " pregnancy and post-pregnancy injuries" more thoroughly. (Ishio Method - Key Principles TM AND Ishio Method – Pelvic Floor Rehab Exercise Protocols TM).

These same concepts apply for our Abdominal Rehabbing...

Ishio Method – Post Pregnancy Rehab Program ™
Terminology:

PF Muscles – Pelvic Floor Muscles
VM Muscle – Vaginal Muscle
Ab Muscles – Abdominal Muscles

Ishio Method – Post Pregnancy Rehab Key Principles ™

*Principle #1: **Core Posture** ™*
*Principle #2: **Surge Posture** ™*
*Principle #3: **Set Posture** ™*
*Principle #4: **Breath Posture** ™*

Principle #1 – Core Posture ™

The ideal pelvis/mid-section position that will have you most efficiently activate and strengthen your PF and Ab muscles during normal daily movements, and fitness exercises. (Ideal Core Box Posture ™),

For example: when you are carrying your groceries - as long as you are standing/moving in an "Ideal Core Box Posture ™", (while utilizing Surge Posture ™), it's as if you are doing formal pelvic floor and abdominal muscle exercises; now imagine this type of benefit, tens of times a day!

This definitely then applies for while you are exercising; because you are moving at a higher intensity while exercising than with "everyday movements", the benefit will also be intensified.

14

Ideal Core Box Posture ™

Ideal Core Box Posture ™ - while standing:

We will talk about how to get into the "Ideal Core Box Posture ™", (as with the photo on the left hand side below), but first, by eliminating the two common incorrect postures that many people use, it will help you more quickly find where the Ideal Core Box Posture ™ is.

In simple terms, you **don't want your pelvis bone overly tucked under/pushed forward**. This is a common standing, carrying, and/or moving hip position of many women who suffer from weak pelvic floor muscles. Many Moms do this when we are carrying our baby on our hip.

"overly tucked/pushed forward"

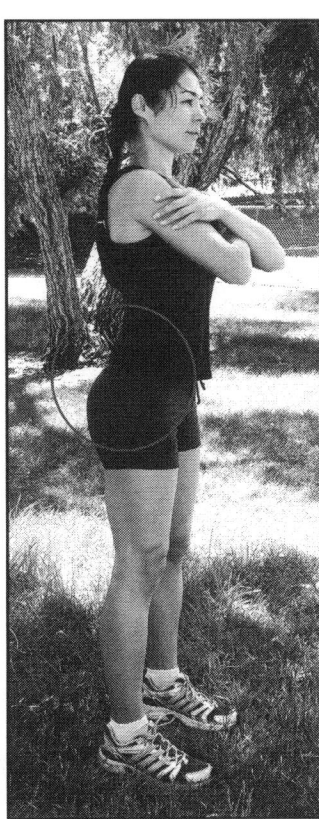 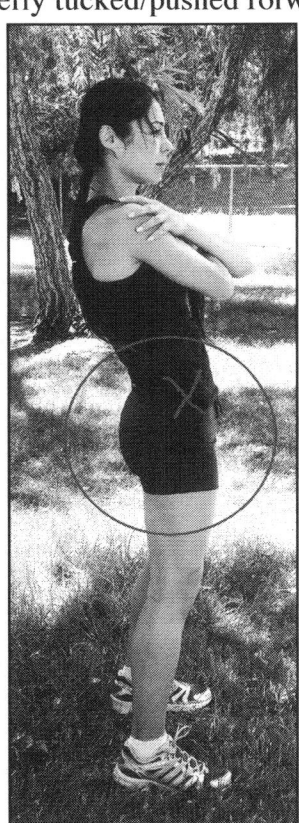

You also don't want your **tailbone overly lifted upwards**, ("butt sticking out far"). This position can usually be indicated by a feeling of pinching or general pain in the lower back after standing for longer periods of time, (and especially after wearing high-heels). For those that usually stand this way, it will make it harder for you to rehab your abdominal muscles, (flatten your "post baby belly"), and lessen any diastasis recti.

(see photos on the next page)

"tailbone overly lifted"

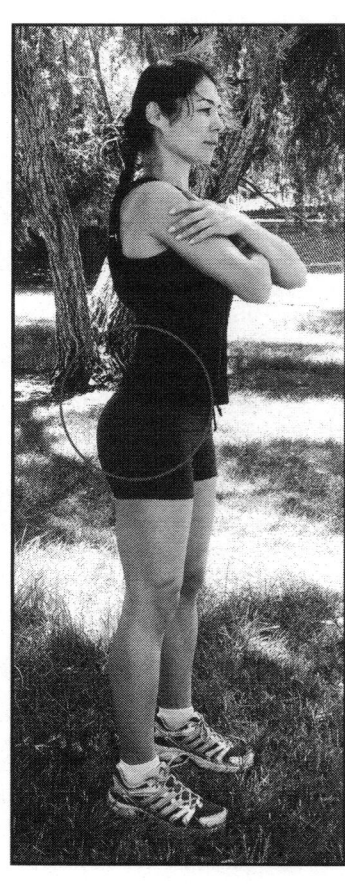

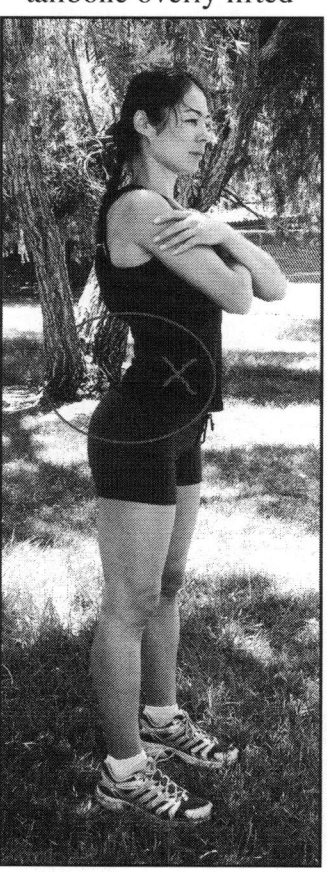

Notice the gap showing, between the tree and the lower back, (right photo), versus the lack of gap in the left photo.

Getting into the Ideal Core Box Posture ™**:** The easiest way for most people to acquaint themselves with how to do this is, to start by standing side-ways next to a mirror. Start by "overly sticking your butt out backwards", (like the photo above on the right), and now slowly **rotate** your pelvis so the bottom of your pelvis bone is rotating slightly forward. You **should feel**, (and when looking in the mirror, you **should see**), your belly button area contract in towards your body, **WHILE** your lower back lengthens/straightens up a bit. *Be sure not to simply push your pelvis area forward incorrectly, (like the photo on the previous page)*.

Keep practicing if you don't get it the first time, most people take many tries.

Ideal Core Box Posture ™ **- during fitness exercises:**

There are many variations of "where" the Ideal Core Box Posture ™ would be during an exercise, and it all depends on what exercise you are doing, or what phase of the exercise you are in, while in motion. Because of this fact, it is not possible to give you one core/hip/pelvis position as a "rule".

One way to ensure that you are in an Ideal Core Box Posture ™ while doing an exercise is to make sure you are doing that exercise correctly.

Example:
When you are standing and about to start a squat, the Ideal Core Box Posture ™ would be that of when you are standing; then as you are going down into your squat, the Ideal Core Box Posture ™ will adjust as you go down. At the bottom phase of a squat, you want to have your hips/butt far back behind you leading the way, with a slight arch in your lower back, allowing your tailbone to have a feeling of lifting slightly upwards. What you don't want is a common mistake with squats, where your knees are leading the way, your lower back is hunching over, and your tailbone is tucking under.

If you do the squat incorrectly, you are doing several things: one, you do NOT have your pelvis/mid-section in an ideal position to effectively strengthen your entire pelvic floor and abdominal muscles; two, your are risking injury to your knees; and three, you are not effectively using the entire length of your quads, (front of your legs), or your hamstrings, (back of legs), or butt, which is the point of the squat exercise.

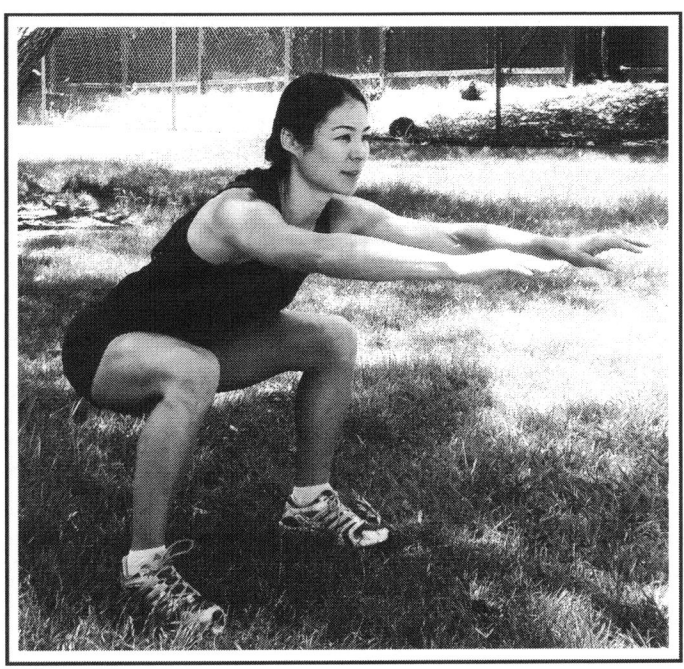

....

Principle #2 – Surge Posture ™

Always contract your pelvic floor and abdominal muscles with 100% efforts, at the SAME TIME, whenever you have short bouts of exertion.

*This WILL help re-train your "muscle reactions".
*This IS doing exercises for your PF and Ab muscles.

Examples of "short bouts of exertion": putting your baby and carrier into the car, when you initially pick up bags of groceries, sneezing, during the exertions phases when you exercise, etc.

We need to re-train our PF and Ab "muscle reactions" after having a baby, and this IS what helps you "re-train" them.

I know this concept is not really known, thought, or talked about, so it's important that we get the word out, so it becomes common knowledge for all women.

Before being pregnant, for most of us, one of two things were happening when we exerted ourselves.

1. We "contracted" our PF and Ab muscles while exerting ourselves…OR
2. We didn't "contract" our PF and Ab muscles while exerting ourselves, but were able to "get away with it", until a pregnancy, surgery, or older age.

If we are having the unconscious default "pushing out/open" muscle reactions during the tens of normal exertions we have throughout the day, those reactions are reinforcing our post-pregnancy muscles with staying weak.

If you have never thought about this concept before, you need to now; even if you had favorable "muscle reactions" before having a baby, it will be "off" after having a baby.

This is especially a negative truth for Moms who are doing what's great and getting in regular exercise, but not having proper "muscle reactions". Exercise requires lots of exertion phases compacted into a short amount of time, so it's even more critical to apply the concept of Surge Posture ™. If you are constantly "pushing out/open" your PF and Ab muscles during exercise, not only are you reinforcing weak muscles as stated above, but possibly you are making it worse.

Again, it is important to do Posture Surges ™ during everyday exertion phases, and especially important every time you exert yourself while exercising.

Think of it this way: when you exert yourself and you don't "contract in" your PF and Ab muscles, then you are probably pushing them "out/open". What will help you maintain discipline is this very real concept, <u>you decide</u>, do you want to "<u>tighten in</u>" or "<u>open out</u>", it's either or, <u>there is no in-between</u>.

Surge Postures ™ are like doing formal PF and Ab specific "exercises"

These are exercises without having to take any extra time out of your schedule, having to have special workout clothes or equipment.

<u>Posture Surges ™ are one of the best "exercises" you can do</u> because anytime you move, it requires core participation, so the simplicity of "pulling-in" your post-pregnancy PF and Ab muscles while you exert yourself throughout the day is like you are continually doing an abdominal exercise to "flatten your stomach", and pelvic floor exercise to strengthen your pelvic floor muscles.

As far as the abdominal muscles are concerned, I call the (Ab) Surge Posture ™ a "walking crunch". In fact, it benefits you better than a plain laying down "crunch" since it's multi-planar, (which basically means that you are moving around in many directions, rather than a one direction up and down crunch). While exerting yourself doing multi-directional tasks and fitness movements, since the movements aren't isolated as a "one directional" movement, you are using your entire "core system" more athletically.

....

Principe #3 – Set Posture ™

Reset the relaxed state of your post pregnancy pelvis floor and abdominal muscles. Throughout the day, maintain roughly 70% of your Surge Posture ™ strength.

<u>It is absolutely normal for women not to remember to maintain Set Posture ™ 100% of the time.</u> Don't worry though, as long as you are consistently applying the other Ishio Method – Post Pregnancy Rehab Key Principles ™, (especially Principles #1 and #2), and doing the Ishio Method – Post Pregnancy Rehab Protocols ™, eventually, maintaining Set Posture ™ will become automatic without you having to think about it at all.

After pregnancy and delivery, the relaxed state with our PF and Ab muscles are not a strong competent part of our "core system"; <u>we need to initially reset our muscles consciously</u>.

Keeping it simple…

Post pregnancy PF and Ab muscles: you want to contract your PF and Ab muscles to about 70% of the strength you are using during a Surge Posture ™, and hold this position for as long as you can remember, (preferably for a few minutes); Do this as often as possible, on and off throughout the entire day.

I say, "for as long as you can remember", because what's normal to happen when doing the Posture Set ™ "exercise" while multi-tasking, without even realizing it, we are back to our post pregnancy relaxed state. The goal is to remember to do this "exercise" many times a day.

Note for you ab muscles: make sure you are only "pulling-in" your Ab muscles to be flush with your body, (not "sucked all the way in"), because you need to be able to properly breathe, (using "diaphragm breathing" – Breath Posture ™).

How far your belly can gently be "pulled in" will of course improve the farther it's been since you've had your baby, AND how properly you've applied the other Ishio Method – Post Pregnancy Rehab Key Principles ™ and Ishio Method – Post Pregnancy Ab Rehab Protocols ™.

………………………………………………………..………………………………………………………

Principle #4 – Breath Posture ™

"Diaphragm breathing" AND Breathing out during exertion

Breathing seems so simple right? We all need to breathe to stay alive, it happens without thinking, so you would think that breathing properly should come naturally on when and how to do it.

Watch how a baby breathes; pretty much all babies properly breathe without restricting their diaphragms. When babies breathe in, their belly "puffs out", and when they breathe out, their belly goes in. For some reason as we get older, we change our breathing habit and start doing the opposite of babies, and do not breathe efficiently anymore.

Let's check how you breathe: Take a deep breath in and pay attention to your belly and pay attention to your chest. Is your chest rising first, (or the most), when you take in a deep breath? Does your belly sit still? Take another deep breath right now to be sure. If you do any of the above mentioned, you are restrictive/shallow breathing.

Many adults breathe with restrictive diaphragms. When you aren't allowing your belly to "puff out" as you breathe in, you aren't allowing your diaphragm to fully drop down, and allowing your lungs/chest cavity to fully expand, and take in a full amount of oxygen.

Diaphragm breathing AND breathing out during exertion phases are very important because remember, <u>our diaphragm is the "top" of our "core rectangle"</u>; by including all sides of our "core rectangle", we will have a more efficient core system, which will help maximize the restoring of our pelvic floor and abdominal muscles.

Properly breathing is also important because then we are getting full oxygen volume into our body, which means clearer thinking, more energy, less stress retention, and easier exercising.

<u>To improve your breathing habit, start breathing like this</u>: You can do this standing up or sitting, but it's the easiest to initially practice while lying down and relaxing the rest of your body.

Put one open hand on your chest, and put the other open hand on your belly button. While taking a deep breathe in, ONLY allow the hand on your belly to rise up first, and then towards the tail end of taking a deep breath, allow your hand on your chest to rise. As you breathe out, your abdominal muscles should contract back in nicely; this is efficient breathing, this is "<u>Diaphragm Breathing</u>". For FYI, diaphragm breathing is something accomplished speakers, singers, dancers, and athletes do.

Golden Rule for Moms

"I AM as IMPORTANT as my children".
Do for ourselves as we do for our children.
It doesn't have to equal the same amount of time,
but it has to equal the same amount of care.

Awareness that you have the ability and responsibility to design the ambiance of your life is powerful wisdom to have; its creativity and productivity are endless.

Chapter Three:

Ishio Method – Pelvic Floor Rehab Exercise Protocol ™

For your use in Chapter 12: Ishio Method – Pelvic Floor Rehab Exercise <u>Check-off Sheets</u>. **Read this chapter to learn and understand the exercises, and then** <u>use the easy check-off sheets as guidance for what you need to do everyday</u>, **and to check your progress.**

Ishio Method – Pelvic Floor Rehab Exercise Protocol's Body Position

Settle Position ™

This body position should be used when doing the morning and evening pelvic floor rehab exercises because it <u>will help keep your entire body relaxed, and allow you to focus on your pelvic area/pelvic floor muscles, while having you in the "Ideal Core Box Position ™"</u>. (Ishio Method Key Principles ™ - Core Posture ™).

While learning/doing "Kegels", many women find themselves contracting muscles that they should not be contracting, (i.e. thighs and buttocks), or having trouble keeping the body relaxed; these issues gets in the way of her being able to focus on how her pelvic floor muscles are feeling, (tightening, relaxing, or moving). *Note: Settle Position ™ is especially important for when being introduced to the rehab exercise during "weeks 11 – 14".*

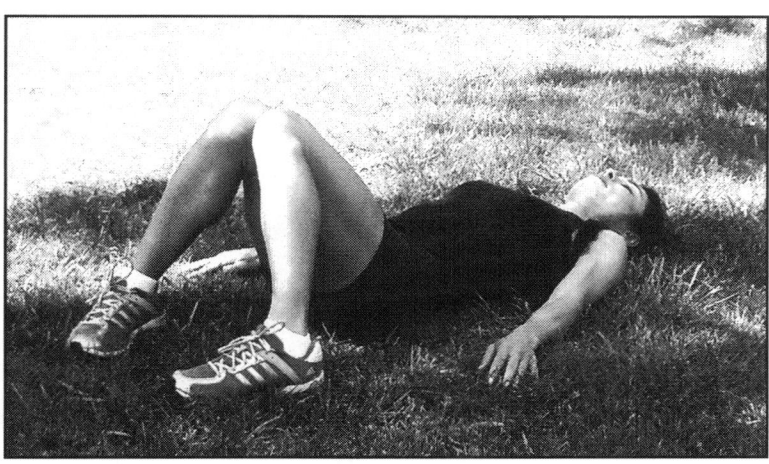

Settle Position TM: Lay on your back. Relax your arms slightly out from the sides of your body. Bend your knees, feet flat, and about shoulder width apart. Slightly turn out your heels as you allow your knees to rest on each other. Lastly, <u>slightly arch your lower-back up</u> from the floor, (you don't want your lower-back flat on the floor, nor do you want an exaggerated arch).

Important practices to slowly introduce with your pelvis floor rehab exercises:
1. Every time you do a pelvic floor muscle exercise, contract your abdominal muscles flush into your body at the same time, (Ab Surge Posture TM).
2. Don't hold your breath during any of the rehab exercises. Also remember, as you take a breath in, you want your belly to "puff out", and as you breathe out, you want your belly to move back into your body, (Breath Posture TM).

1st week through 3rd week

Introducing: <u>Endurance Technique</u> TM

As the name says, this technique will build muscle strength and endurance for the rest of the Ishio Method - Pelvic Floor Rehab Exercise Protocol TM.

Endurance Technique: Contract your PF muscles, (a "traditional Kegel"), and hold for "one bout". One bout is contracting as hard as you can, for as long as you can.

The reasons why I say, "as long as you can", rather than having a specific time, are for several reasons:

1. At the beginning phase, you don't want the pressure or limit of there being a "right or wrong" amount of time. The main thing is to do it consistently with appropriate effort, throughout the day.
2. We should in general, have a "pulled in/up" posture with our pelvic floor muscles at all times; especially after delivering a baby vaginally, we are in immediate need to re-calibrate this vital posture. (Set Posture TM)

Goal - Endurance Technique TM**:**
3 sets of "as long as you can", (first thing in the morning, last thing at bedtime), and 1 set during the day, (where noted on the next page).

When to do the Endurance Technique ᴛᴍ:
(remember to use the "check-off sheets" as reference)

1. Right after waking up in the morning (while still laying down):
You have been in a state of relaxation all night, and you need a PF muscles morning "re-set".
3 sets.
2. Right after using the toilet: You need to reinforce the "pulling in and upward" posture once again. 1 set of 10 seconds.
3. At the start of feeding your baby: 1 set.
4. At the start of changing your baby's diaper: 1 set.
5. Before going to bed (while laying down): 3 sets.

Reminders: Ishio Method - Post Pregnancy Rehab Key Principles ᴛᴍ

When exerting yourself by putting the baby and carrier into your car, etc, make sure you contract "in" both the PF and Ab muscles, (Surge Posture ᴛᴍ), as you breathe out, (Breath Posture ᴛᴍ).

Whenever you are walking: Keep you pelvis/mid-section in the ideal position, (Core Posture ᴛᴍ), so you can get the maximum benefit with toning your Ab and PF muscles during regular movements, AND for accelerating improvements with Set Posture ᴛᴍ.

****

4ᵗʰ week through 6ᵗʰ week

* Make habit, the Ishio Method – Post Pregnancy Rehab Key Principles ᴛᴍ
* Continue Endurance Technique ᴛᴍ

Introducing: Pulse Technique ᴛᴍ

Pulse Technique ᴛᴍ: Contract, (pull in/up), your PF muscles until you are at "100% pulled-in", and hold for roughly a count of 2, then slowly relax your PF muscles, (but don't relax more than 50% from being completely relaxed), then re-contract…this is one revolution.

Goal – Pulse Technique ™:
1 set = 10 revolutions in a row.

When to do the Pulse Technique ™: *(remember to use the "check-off sheets" as reference)*

1. <u>In the morning after waking up</u> (while still laying down): Do 1 set of Endurance Technique ™, then do 2 sets of Pulse Technique ™.
2. <u>During the afternoon</u>: Do the Endurance Technique ™ after using the toilet, at the start of feeding your baby, at the start of changing your baby's diaper.
 3. <u>In the evening before going to bed</u>: Do 1 set of Endurance Technique ™, then do 2 sets of Pulse Technique ™.

****

7th week through 10th week

* Make habit, the Ishio Method – Post Pregnancy Rehab Key Principles ™
* Continue Endurance Technique ™ and Pulse Technique ™

Introducing: Anti-Gravity Position ™ and Popins Technique ™

Introducing: Anti-Gravity Position ™

Use gravity to your advantage.

Anti-Gravity Position ™: Lie down on the floor, put pillows under your hips so they are raised off the floor a few inches; have your legs relax on a chair, seat of a sofa, or side of a bed.

After delivering a baby, your VM muscle is the weakest of the PF muscles. Gravity and the weight of our organs make rehabbing the VM muscles, (also Ab muscles) more challenging. With that said, we want to have an opportunity to give those muscles a break from the effects of gravity when initially rehabilitating our VM/PF/Ab muscles.

Important Note: Those with C-sections, (or other pelvis, lower-back, or pain issues of the like), will need to wait until after clearance from your doctor to use the Anti-Gravity Position ™. This is a recommendation for normal, healthy individuals. It is also your personal choice in regards to continuing the Anti-Gravity Position ™ after the 12-week mark.

When to use the Anti-Gravity Position тм:

1. At the end of the day: Evening is a good time for the Anti-Gravity Position тм since gravity has created pressure on your body throughout the day, and you have the space to do it at home.

Introducing: Popins Technique тм

Popins Technique тм: Contract your PF as "pulled-in/up" as you can for a fraction of a second, then immediately relax up to 50% of our relaxed state, (and for only a fraction of a second), and repeat. Basically it's a "pop" contract in, to a fraction of a second relax, and back to a "pop" contract in, and repeat.

Goal – Popins Technique тм:
1 set = 10 revolutions in a row.

When to do the Popins Technique тм: *(remember to use the "check-off sheets" as reference)*

1. In the morning after waking up (while still laying down): Do 1 set of Endurance Technique тм, 1 set of Pulse Technique тм, 2 sets of the Popins Technique тм.
2. During the afternoon: Do the Endurance Technique тм after using the toilet, at the start of feeding your baby, at the start of changing your baby's diaper.
3. In the evening before going to bed (while laying down): Do 1 set of Endurance Technique тм, 1 set of Pulse Technique тм, and 2 sets of Popins Technique тм, (in Anti-Gravity Position тм if you can or choose to).

* During intercourse. (This is for when you eventually start having sex again). Practice for a few minutes at the beginning, (along with the Endurance Technique тм, and Pulse Technique тм).

For the rest of the "session", always maintain Set Posture тм, (maintaining at least "70%" of your "100%" contracting effort of your PF muscles), and as you feel, sporadically add in Surge Postures тм, (contracting to 100% effort of your PF muscles). **Doing these will accelerate your improvements with your mind-body connection for your rehab exercises, gives your muscles resistance, and also improves sex life.**

"Exercises" during intercourse are not noted on the "check-off sheets", but don't forget this because this will accelerate your improvements.

****

11th week through 14th week

* Make habit, the Ishio Method – Post Pregnancy Rehab Key Principles ™
* Continue Endurance Technique ™, Pulse Technique ™, and Popins Technique ™

Introducing: Iso-Form ™

With the Iso-Form ™, you will be contracting the <u>entire length</u> of the VM muscle, (with the strongest point being the middle), rather than the entire PF muscles, (as with the other rehab exercises so far, or with the "Kegels" as we are commonly doing them).

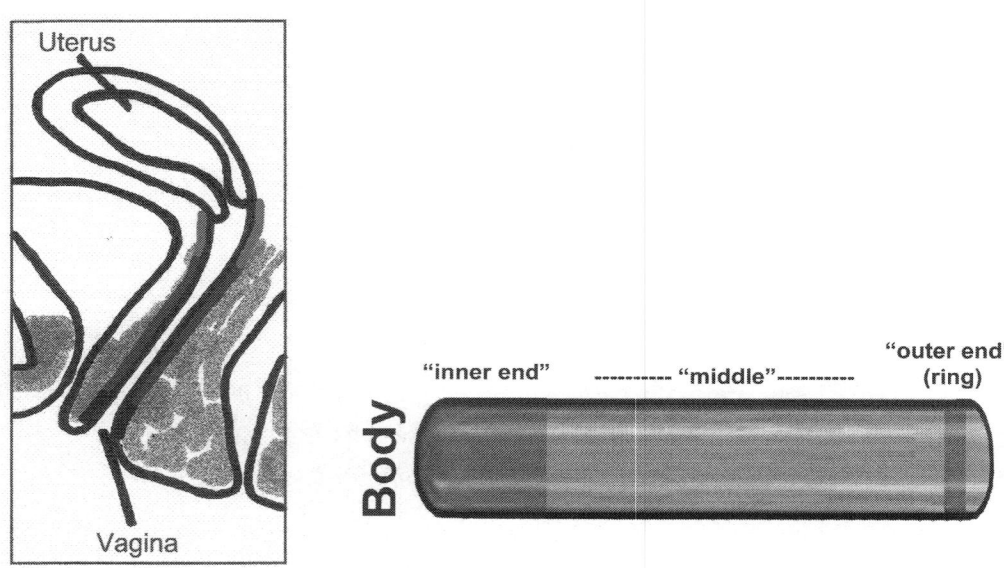

The reason why it's important to learn to isolate the VM muscle is because when doing "traditional kegels", you are activating the entire PF muscle's "basket", and are not targeting the entire length of the VM muscle in a way that post pregnancy Moms can get the best benefit.

As well, although the Ishio Method – Post Pregnancy Rehab Key Principles ™ are extremely critical with post-pregnancy recovery, the Iso-Form ™ is an exceptionally effective addition that is direct/precise with helping strengthen, re-lengthen, and make more dense, the part of the PF muscle group that was the most affected with pregnancy, (especially after vaginal delivery).

The mind body connection that you attain is another big plus with this rehab exercise because it significantly enhances sex life.

Note: When isolating the VM muscle using the Iso-Form ™, you will still be activating your other PF muscles; however, the obvious emphasis in contraction will be the length of the VM muscle.

Important: Don't worry if the Iso-Form ™ is not "perfected" by the end of the 14th week; these weeks are simply the weeks the Iso-Form ™ is being introduced. <u>It is not expected for you to be completely proficient with this technique within these weeks</u>. It takes most women the entire length of the rehab program, (many times longer), before they feel like they are having more ease with the mind-body connection necessary to isolate the VM muscle.

On another note: even after you achieve the mind-body connection with the Iso-Form ™, <u>it is normal to not have much strength when doing them initially</u>. It takes time to gain enough control to where you can start focusing on the strength of the Iso-Form ™.

Getting Started With Iso-Form ™

The best thing for all women and Moms is to simply know that it is possible.

Feel:

When "isolating" the VM Muscle, it will have a different feel then when doing any of the other Ishio Method ™ – Pelvic Floor Rehab exercises so far, (or the "traditional kegels").

Instead of a "pulling in/up" or a "balling up" feeling, you will have more of the feeling of "flattening" the sides of the VM muscle "walls" together.

Visualize:

Open both of your hands as straight as you can, while keeping all of your fingers together so there are no spaces between them. Now put your hands together, and match your palm to palm and fingers to fingers together. Press your hands and fingers together, evenly distributing the strength of the "press"; this is what the Iso-Form ™ should feel like, versus the "balling into a fist" feeling you get with the other exercises.

While you are improving your mind-body connection for the Iso-Form ™, it should help to visualize your open palms/fingers pressing against each other.

Use The Settle Position ™ When Learning To Activate Iso-Form ™

Refer back to the beginning of this chapter; there is a photo and detailed description for the Settle Position ™.

Tips on how to "activate" Iso-Form ™:

1. Do a "body check" and make sure your entire body is relaxed.

2. Do the Endurance Technique ™ and hold for 15 seconds.

3. Gradually relax you PF muscles, (but only up to a 50% relaxed state), and then "re-tighten" slowly, (while concentrating on the "balling-pulling in/up" feeling. Do this a few times.

4. Now on to the Iso-Form ™: on the next "re-tightening" phase, don't "tighten" to 100% like you have been so far, (since you are simply trying to learn the mind-body connection at this point). Keep the "tightening" very light in strength, and visualize "flattening" as with the "two hands pressing together" example I gave you earlier. Even if you aren't sure you are doing it correctly, hold for 10 seconds.

5. Now alternate between doing the Endurance Technique ™, (and concentrating on the "balling-pulling up/in" feeling), and the Iso-Form ™, (and concentrate on a "flattening" feeling); you will eventually feel a slight difference, and can reference from there.

Still Having A Hard Time With The Mind-Body Connection For The Iso-Form ™, There Are "Reference Tools" That Can Help

Despite using a "reference tool", many will initially still be contracting the entire PF muscles rather than isolating the VM muscle, but at least with a "reference tool", it will get you faster on your way to improved mind-body connection; by allowing you to better be able to "feel" the contracting of your VM muscle, versus your entire PF muscles.

I will start by introducing the simplest, most "organic", option first.

#1. Your partner during sex:

This will give you a "reference point" for better mind-body connection for the Iso-Form ™ exercises, as well, it will give you isometric resistance to help tone your VM muscle.

Directions:

To improve mind-body connection, during intercourse, ask your partner to hold still, and do the Endurance Technique TM, and Iso-Form Technique TM exercises for a couple minutes.

Important Tip Reminder: for isometric resistance during sex, to help tone and strengthen your muscles, always maintain Set Posture TM, (maintain at least 70% tautness of your PF muscles), and as you feel, add in Surge Postures TM, (contracting to 100% tautness of your PF muscles); do this throughout the entire session, every time.

You don't have to worry about it "being weird"; the fact of the matter is, doing these exercises drastically improves the experience for BOTH partners, and your VM muscle "control" will drastically improve as well.

PLEASE NOTE Before Moving Forward: for the purpose of rehabbing your post-pregnancy PF/VM muscles, if the only "reference tool" or "toning device" of your choice is your partner during sex, (because the other options contained after this section are simply not for you), that is a perfectly fine decision; when you properly follow the Ishio Method – Post-Pregnancy Rehab Principles and Protocols TM, you will have very successful improvements regardless.

#2. A simple thin no-thrills dildo:

(You want the diameter of the apparatus to be minimal, because you want to "flatten" your VM muscle as close to each other as possible).

Directions: Lay down on a firm surface, (in the Settle Position TM), and simply alternate between practicing the Endurance Technique TM, and the Iso-Form TM, using this "reference tool".

IMPORTANT NOTE: the types of "Toning Devices" that will be mentioned on the next page are **NOT** meant for specifically learning to isolate contraction of the VM muscle, (Iso-Form TM). The reason why I am mentioning them in this section is because these are options available for women who want more resistance with their PF muscles training, so I am sharing this information.

As noted above, if you feel that these "Toning Devices" are simply not for you, that is a perfectly fine decision; when you properly follow the Ishio Method – Post-Pregnancy Rehab Principles and Protocols TM, you will have very successful improvements regardless.

IMPORTANT NOTE: <u>I am **Not Endorsing** any of these "Toning Devices". I have never used any of them, nor have any of my clients ever used them.</u> The options are being noted because they are available for women, and I would like to share the information.

Toning Devices

These "toning devices" are good for if you would like to add resistance with your PF muscles training.

Please note that there have not been any wide/objective studies conducted on the actual benefits/risks of these "devices".

Gyneflex:
This is an apparatus that's made of a plastic material. From a quick and simple description, it is shaped like big tweezers, with the angular end to be inserted into your vagina. Basically you squeeze the "tweezers" with your vagina, and that act will strengthen your VM/PF muscles. They offer three resistances. Cost is about $40.

Vagina Weights, (i.e. Aquaflex, Kegel Exercise Weights):
(For those who want to increase their PF/ VM muscles "strength". With these types of apparatus', you have flexibility with how much weight you want to add to the exercise).

Aquaflex: You insert a part of the apparatus into your vagina, (they call it a cone), then add weights to the rope type attachment that extends from the "cone", (that hangs externally from your body). The goal is to keep the cone from falling out of your body.

Kegel Exercise Weights: You insert cone shaped weight into your vagina, and the goal is to keep it from falling out; there are assortments of different weights.

For both types of "weights", as you improve your PF muscle's strength, you go up to a heavier weight. Cost is about $50 – $60.

* There are other "toning device" options available, but listed above are the basic kinds *

Important Note: discontinue use of any apparatus if you are in pain, and seek further medical advice.

Goal – Iso-Form ᴛᴍ:
3 sets of holding for 5 seconds.
Increase the time by 5 seconds until you reach sets of 15 seconds.
The goal also is for fluidity between contracting your VM and PF Muscles.

When to do the Iso-Form ᴛᴍ: *(remember to use the "check-off sheets" as reference)*

1. In the morning after waking up (while still laying down): Do 1 set of Endurance Technique ᴛᴍ, 1 set of Pulse Technique ᴛᴍ. Then using Iso-Form ᴛᴍ, (emphasizing the VM muscle), do 1 set Endurance Technique ᴛᴍ, *(remember, in Settle Position ᴛᴍ)*.
2. During the afternoon: Do the Endurance Technique ᴛᴍ after using the toilet, at the start of feeding your baby, at the start of changing your baby's diaper.
3. In the evening before going to bed (while laying down): Do 1 set Endurance Technique ᴛᴍ, and 2 sets Popins Technique ᴛᴍ. Then using Iso-Form ᴛᴍ, (emphasizing the VM muscle), do 2 sets Endurance Technique ᴛᴍ, *(remember, in Settle Position ᴛᴍ)*.

* During intercourse. (This is for when you eventually start having sex again). Practice for a few minutes at the beginning, (along with the Endurance and Pulse Technique ᴛᴍ).

For the rest of the "session", always maintain Set Posture ᴛᴍ, (maintaining at least "70%" of your "100%" contracting effort of your PF muscles), and as you feel, sporadically add in Surge Postures ᴛᴍ, (contracting to 100% effort of your PF muscles). **Doing these will accelerate your improvements with your mind-body connection for your rehab exercises, gives your muscles resistance, and also improves sex life.**

"Exercises" during intercourse are not noted on the "check-off sheets", but don't forget this because this will accelerate your improvements.

When you are able to easily "activate" Iso-Form ᴛᴍ with the Endurance Technique ᴛᴍ, then you can move on to the next section

Note: There are many women who stay in the Iso-Form Technique ᴛᴍ "phase" longer than the designated 11th – 14th week plan. It is OK to stay in this "phase" longer; it will not negatively affect your post pregnancy rehab success AS LONG AS you are regularly implementing the Ishio Method – Post Pregnancy Rehab Key Principles ᴛᴍ and continue doing the Ishio Method – Pelvic Floor Rehab Protocol ᴛᴍ up to this point.

****

15th week through 16th week

* Make habit, the Ishio Method – Post Pregnancy Rehab Key Principles ™
* Continue grasping the Iso-Form ™
* Continue Endurance Technique ™, Pulse Technique ™, and Popins Technique ™

Adding: Pulse Technique WITH Iso-Form ™

Goal - The goal is to gain even better mind-body connection with isolating the VM muscle, and gaining more strength, making more dense, the entire VM muscle's length.

When to do the Pulse Technique WITH Iso-Form ™:
(remember to use the "check-off sheets" as reference)

1. In the morning after waking up (while still laying down): Do 2 sets of Popins Technique ™. Then WITH Iso-Form ™, do 1 set Endurance Technique ™, and 1 set Pulse Technique ™.
2. During the afternoon: Do the Endurance Technique ™ after using the toilet, at the start of feeding your baby, at the start of changing your baby's diaper.
3. In the evening before going to bed (while laying down): Do 1 set Endurance Technique ™. Then WITH Iso-Form ™, do 1 set Endurance Technique ™, and 2 sets Pulse Technique ™.

* During intercourse. (This is for when you eventually start having sex again). Practice for a few minutes at the beginning, (along with the Endurance and Pulse Technique ™).

For the rest of the "session", always maintain Set Posture ™, (maintaining 70% of your "100%" contracting effort of your PF muscles), and sporadically add in Surge Postures ™, (contracting to 100% effort of your PF muscles). **Doing these will accelerate your improvements with your mind-body connection for your rehab exercises, gives your muscles resistance, and also improves sex life.**

CONGRATULATIONS!
You have completed the Ishio Method - Pelvic Floor Rehab Exercise Protocol ™

It is critical for your continued improvements, and long-term maintenance, that you continue doing pelvis floor exercises. On the next page is a maintenance protocol; follow the principles daily, and do the exercises a few times a week.

Ishio Method ™ - Pelvic Floor Rehab Maintenance Protocol ™

Main Principles
• Core Posture TM
• Surge Posture TM
• Set Posture TM
• Breathe Posture TM

Set Posture TM and Surge Posture TM

- While Exercising
- During Intercourse

Endurance Technique TM

- Right after using the toilet. (5 seconds)

Mornings: (in bed)

1 set	Endurance Technique TM		30 seconds
1 set	Popins Technique TM		10 count

Throughout Day:

Apply the Ishio Method - Post Pregnancy Key Principles TM

Do random Ishio Method - Post Pregnancy Rehab Pelvic Floor Exercises TM

Before Bed: (in bed)

1 set	Endurance Technique TM		30 seconds
1 set	Pulse Technique TM		10 count

Reminders:

By maintaining proper Core Posture TM, and doing Surge Postures TM throughout the day when doing "normal" activities, you will automatically be helping maximize the toning of your PF muscles.

Through conscious Surge Posture TM practice, eventually, whenever exerting yourself, your PF muscles will have an "automatic reaction" of contracting "in/up", without having to think about it.

As your PF/VM muscles increase in density, you will require much less thoughts or efforts with maintaining Set Posture TM throughout everyday living.

Optional Extra Credit

Only once you have <u>successfully completed the Ishio Method - Pelvic Floor Rehab Exercise Protocol ™, and also gained ease and ability with the Iso-Form ™,</u> are you probably ready to move to this more intricate exercise.

<u>The reason I call this "Extra Credit" is because you don't need to be able to do this in order to have a COMPLETE and SUCCESSFUL post-pregnancy rehab of your PF/VM muscles, or for general pelvic floor health. If at this point you choose this is not for you, then that is a 100% correct choice for you.</u>

The main purpose of the "Extra Credit" would be strictly for personal preference of expanded mind-body connection, and additional confidence with your body awareness, and/or enhancing your sex life.

Ishio Method - Extra Credit

"Ishio Method ™ – Extra Credit" is having the ability to isolate the emphasis of where you are contracting your VM muscle, and the fluidity of transferring emphasis from once "area" to another.

Note: A woman is able to contract the VM muscle with emphasis with the "outer end", the "middle" (the entire length), and the "inner end" of the VM muscle.

Don't let the sentence you just read seem overwhelming. Being able to do the Iso-Form ™ IS already being able to emphasize the "middle", and being able to do the Endurance Technique ™ is being able to emphasize the "outer end".

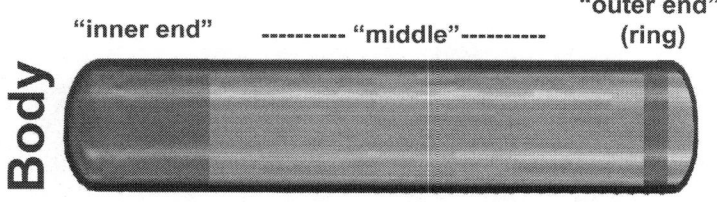

Learning How To Do The "Ishio Method ™ - Extra Credit"

The best way to learn this, first and foremost, is by simply knowing it is possible.

The second way is to be very proficient with the Ishio Method – Post Pregnancy Rehab Protocol ™ techniques that we have already been doing.

The next way is to have a reference point. A reference point would be very helpful with the speed at which you can gain enough mind/body connection, hence, the recommendation of "practicing" during sex, as we talked about in the Iso-Form ™ section of the Ishio Method – Post Pregnancy Rehab Protocol ™.

Final advice is to use "visualization" to improve mind/body control. You can decide what that "visualization" needs to be for yourself.

Step 1

Start with what you already know how to do

"Outer-end"
Again, as mentioned before, doing the Endurance Technique ™ is the "outer end" of the VM muscle. Practice the Endurance Technique ™ and pay attention to how it feels as you tighten, then release.

"Middle"
The Iso-Form ™ IS contracting the "middle".

As talked about before, it is a "flattening" feeling, (not a "pulling in" or "balling up" feeling), as with the commonly known "Kegels". Now practice the Iso-Form ™ and pay attention to how the "flattening" feeling feels in comparison to the "balling up" feeling of the Endurance Technique ™.

Step 2

Do the Endurance Technique ™, then slowly release, then immediately go do the Iso-Form ™, and repeat.

Pay attention to the differences with the feeling of "pulling in/balling up", and then "flattening". Keep trying this until you can easily and smoothly transition back and forth.

Step 3

"Inner"…this step will probably be the most challenging for most.

Until you are very proficient with Step 1 and Step 2, and transitioning very easily and smoothly between "outer" and "middle", I would recommend waiting on going on to Step 3.

Unlike the "flattening" feeling with Iso-Form TM, or the strong "pulling-in/balling up" feeling of the Endurance Technique TM, contracting the "inner section" will be more of subtle "pinching/squeezing" feeling.

This last step is all about visualization and experimenting until you figure out what it takes for you to engage the mind/body connection it takes to contract the "inner-end". As far as visualization, that is up to what visualization works for you.

Other Tips To Get You On Your Way With The "Inner-end"

* Having a "reference tool", (as we spoke about with the Iso-Form TM), will give you a much needed reference that you most likely will initially need for the mind-body connection. You will gain the ability much faster, and once you have the mind-body connection, you won't need the "reference tool" anymore.

* Start with Iso-Form TM, (contracting the "middle"), and with only releasing a tad, slowly try to contract the "inner end". This is where it requires visualization, (as with the "reference tool"), and you want to visualize as you are transitioning to contracting the "inner section".

At the beginning, probably nothing will happen, but keep visualizing; eventually something very subtle will happen. It's so subtle that you may think, "does that count?", but that is the start of the mind/body connection you need. The rest is up to you as far as practicing and making that subtle movement become more pronounced and stronger.

Finally

Once you have ease with the "outer to middle" and the "middle to inner", then you can start practicing going continuously through from the "outer end", all the way through the "inner end" and vice versa. At first it will probably be "blocky" movements, then with practice, it will become more of a roll.

Chapter Four:

Ishio Method - Abdominal Rehab Exercise Protocol ™

For your use in Chapter 12: Ishio Method – Abdominal Rehab Exercise <u>Check-off Sheets</u>. Read this chapter to learn and understand the exercises, and then <u>use the easy check-off sheets as guidance for what you need to do everyday</u>, and to check your progress.

1ˢᵗ week

Wear your Sillo Belly Wrap ™ while you sleep at night, and during part of the day; throughout the day, give your skin about 30 minute breather breaks here and there.

Start acquainting yourself with Ishio Method – Post Pregnancy Rehab Key Principles ™; Core Posture ™, Surge Posture ™, Set Posture ™, and Breath Posture ™.

****

2ⁿᵈ Week through 4ᵗʰ Week

* *Make habit, Ishio Method – Post Pregnancy Rehab Key Principles ™*
**Continue wearing the* <u>*Sillo Belly Wrap ™*</u> *at night while you sleep, (crossing in front)*

Introducing: Seated Pull-ins ™

Re-calibrate your mind-body connection with your abdominal muscles. Gently pull the two halves of your "six-pack" together, and start flattening your stomach.

Seated Pull-ins ™:
Note: you can do this standing up too; just make sure you are standing with Core Posture ™ in mind.

1. Sit in a sturdy chair.

2. Make sure you are sitting up tall with your shoulders drawn "back and down" for good upper-body posture.

3. Take a deep breath in. Reminder: Breath Posture ™ – allow your belly to move out a tad as you breathe in.

Note: you only need to very partially relax your belly "out" while you breathe in, (because post-pregnancy bellies are especially lax), and it easily "opens up" enough to allow the diaphragm to "drop" freely, enabling you to get in a deep proper breath.

4. <u>As you breathe out slowly, slowly pull-in your abdominal muscles as far in as you can, and hold for a couple seconds.</u>

5. Repeat 7 times.

Advancing:

If you would like a bit more of a challenge, then get on your hands and knees, and do this same exercise in that position. Reminder: when on your hands and knees, don't lock your arms, and remember to have your shoulders drawn back, (and not hunched towards your ears).

Goal – Seated Pull-ins ™:

1 set at a time - 7 repetitions per set

Several sets throughout the day, (right before every meal, when driving, standing in line, when watching TV, etc.)

<u>**2nd week – 4th week:**</u> *(remember to use the "check-off sheets" as reference)*

Daily – At least 5 sets of Seated Pull-ins ™

<u>CAUTION: Before moving onto the next phases, you must check to see where your "diastasis recti" level is</u>

What Is Diastasis Recti?

Our abdominal wall is compromised of many different directions of muscles. The muscles that we need to check about for Diastasis Recti is the muscle that we commonly refer to as our "six-pack".

When you look at a "six-pack", you will notice that there is a space that splits the "six-pack" from a left side and a right side. When you are pregnant and your belly grows, that space gets much wider apart. After you are done being pregnant, that split doesn't automatically come back together as it was before; it is a slower process that takes a little time.

If a woman starts exerting her abdominal muscles too aggressively before that space has a chance to close up enough, (by doing too heavy lifting, "sit-ups", or of the like), then she will run the risk of not having that space come together properly, or even making the space wider apart. When the space is too wide apart, this can lead to many ailments such as a hernia, lower back pain, and the appearance of a still pregnant belly, to name a few.

How To Check To See If Your Abs Are At A Safer Position

Lay down on the ground, on your back, with your knees bent, and your feet flat on the floor. Now slightly lift your head/shoulders of the ground, (just enough so you are flexing your abdominal muscle), and feel the space in between both halves of your "six-pack". The ideal space in between both sides of the "six-pack" muscles is to have it no more than two finger width apart, (the index and middle finger).

If you haven't passed the "two finger test", don't worry; you just may simply need a little more time. Don't be overly concerned with needing to rush more difficult abdominal exercises right away because if your diastasis recti space stays the same or gets worse, you can end up needing surgery.

If you have significant "diastasis recti", wait a few more weeks, and re-check before moving forward. Continue doing the Seated Pull-ins ᴛᴍ, and wearing your Sillo Belly Wrap ᴛᴍ.

If you are around the two-finger width mark, proceed with caution by paying precise attention to the "Abdominal Exercise Posture" described on the next page.

Important: "Abdominal Exercise Posture"

It is very important that you maintain proper "Abdominal Exercise Posture" when doing any of these rehab exercises; think Surge Posture ™, ("pulling in" your abdominal muscles while you are exerting yourself).

When not keeping proper "Abdominal Exercise Posture" during these ab exercises, you will be "pushing out" your abdominal muscles, which is contradictory to what your goal is. Also it risks your abdominal separation with taking longer to improve, or even getting worse.

Important: Progression From One Abdominal Exercise To The Next

The way you ultimately know when you can progress from one level to the next level is by your ability, and not by the "weeks" noted in the Ishio Method – Post Pregnancy Ab Rehab Protocol ™. If you need to spend an extra week or two on a specific exercise/level, then simply do that; in the long run, it will benefit your ability for the more difficult exercises later on, and keep your abdominal/core area safe.

****

5th Week through 8th Week

* Make habit, Ishio Method – Post Pregnancy Rehab Key Principles ™
*Continue wearing the <u>Sillo Belly Wrap</u> ™ at night while you sleep, (crossing in front)
*Continue doing the Seated Pull-ins ™

Introduction: Incline Planks ™
Improve total core strength; including upper body strength, and posture.

Incline Planks ™:

1. Use a sofa, bench, or chair.
2. While standing, pull-in your abdominal muscles tightly.
3. Start by placing your hands on the part you sit. Extend one leg out at a time, and go into a "push-up" position.
4. Re-check to make sure that your Ab muscles are in a "pulled-in" position. Make sure to draw your shoulders back, and open your chest for good upper back posture. Also make sure you are not "locking" your arms, and are keeping your hips from "drooping down".

5. Do 3 sets of 20 seconds.

Incline Planks

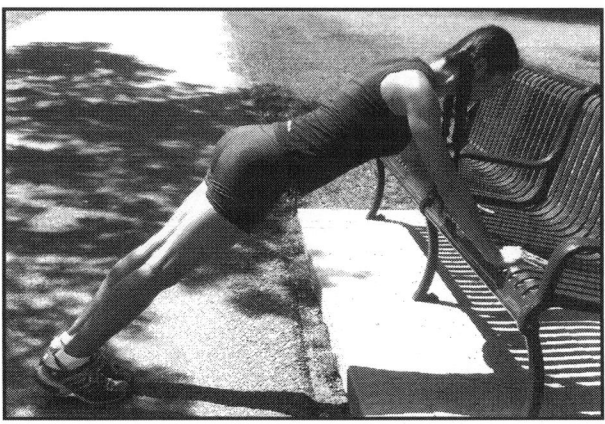

<u>Advancing:</u>
Start adding increments of 5 seconds, until your reach 45 seconds.

Goal - Incline Planks ™:
1 time a day - 3 sets of 45 seconds

Note: Slight protruding belly is normal when doing these right after having a baby, but you should feel the tension of your muscle <u>pulling into your spine at all times</u>.

Info to know:*For many people, what's the most focused on during "planks" are with keeping the hips "up off the ground", (from drooping), but often times, the shoulders/upper back posture is neglected. What I want you to also focus on is with keeping your upper-back pulled back and chest opened.*

Planks are hard, so curling the shoulders forward is a natural reaction by our body trying to do anything it can to help keep our hips "off the ground". Imagine standing with this same curled over "bad" posture; definitely something we don't want, so it's important to not reinforce this posture while doing exercises.

5th week – 8th week: *(remember to use the "check-off sheets" as reference)*
Once Daily – 3 sets of Incline Planks ™, several sets of Seated Pull-ins ™

****

9th Week through 13th Week

* Make habit, Ishio Method – Post Pregnancy Rehab Key Principles TM
*Continue wearing the <u>Sillo Belly Wrap</u> TM at night while you sleep, (<u>at 13-weeks, cross in back</u>)
*Continue doing the Seated Pull-ins TM

Two exercises: <u>Standing Tilts</u> TM *and Half and Half Planks TM*

Introduction: Standing Tilts TM

Gently pulling the two halves of your "six-pack" together, and flattening the stomach.

Standing Tilts TM:

1. Stand with "good posture", *(chapter 6, pages 71 & 79)*, and feet shoulder width apart.
2. Place hands on your hips.
3. Now pull your abdominal muscles into your body <u>as tightly as you can</u>; this is important so you aren't letting your belly pop out.
4. <u>Slightly</u> lean your hips forward for a second, (see photo below), then go back to the starting "good posture" for a second; and repeat 10 times. Continually re-check that your <u>abs are being pulled in tightly the entire time</u>.

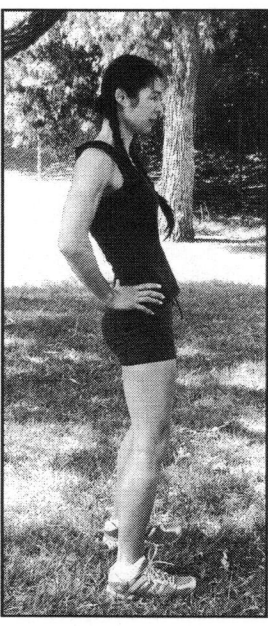

Goal - Standing Curls TM:
1 time a day - 2 sets of 15 pulse repetitions

Introduction: Half and Half Planks TM

These will replace the Incline Planks TM. Improve total core strength, including upper body strength, and posture.

Half and Half Planks TM:

1. Kneel on the floor, onto your hands and knees.
2. Pull-in your abdominal muscles as tightly as you can.
3. Come down onto your forearm to hold up your body, (and make sure your elbows are directly below your shoulders).
4. Extend one leg out. *Important Note: you want the emphasis of your "weight" on the leg that's extended, so it is doing most of the strength work.*
5. Re-check that your abdominal muscles are "pulled-in", that you have "good upper body posture", (shoulders drawn back, chest opened), and your hips are not "drooping down".

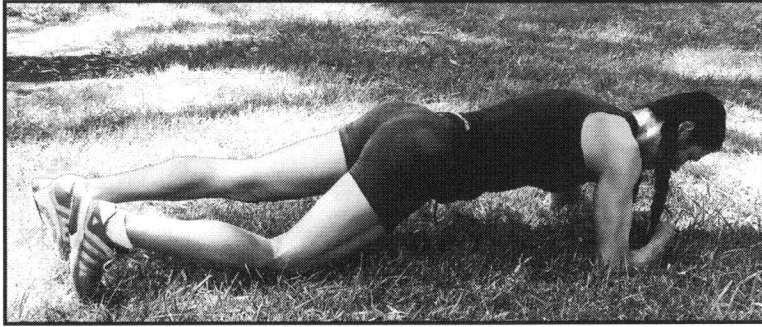

5. Hold for 10 seconds, then switch leg positions, (extend the other leg that was just bent, and bend the leg that was just extended).
6. Do 3 sets.

Advancing: Start adding increments of 5 seconds until you reach 20 seconds on each side.

Goal - Half and Half Planks TM:
1 time a day - 3 sets of 20 seconds on each side

Info to remember: Planks are hard, so curling the shoulders forward is a natural reaction by our body trying to do anything it can to help keep our hips off the ground. Imagine standing with this same curled over "bad" posture; definitely something we don't want, so it's important to not reinforce this posture while doing exercises.

9th week – 13th week: *(remember to use the "check-off sheets" as reference)*
Once Daily – 2 sets of Standing Tilt TM, 3 sets of Half and Half Planks TM

****

14th Week through 17th Week

* *Make habit, Ishio Method – Post Pregnancy Rehab Key Principles TM*
**Continue wearing the <u>Sillo Belly Wrap</u> TM at night while you sleep, (crossing in the back)*
**Continue doing the Half and Half Planks TM*

Two exercises: *Micro-Crunches TM and Toe Taps TM*

Introduction: Micro-Crunches TM

Gently pulling the two halves of your "six-pack" together, and flattening the stomach.

Micro-Crunches TM:

1. Lay on the floor, onto your back; bend your knees, and only have the heels of your feet on the floor.
2. Press your lower back into the floor, and pull-in your abdominal muscles tightly. *Note: maintain this position the entire time you are doing this exercise.*
3. Lift your shoulders off the floor as high as you can comfortably go without lifting your lower back off the floor, and hold; <u>this is your "starting position".</u>

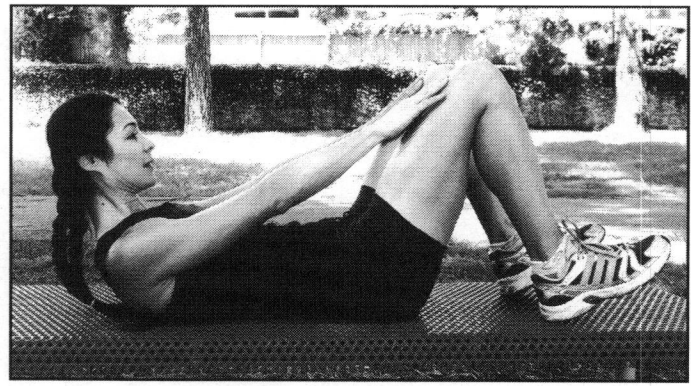

4. Re-check to make sure your lower back is still pressed into the floor, and your abs are pulled-in tightly.

5. Now, leading with your shoulders, <u>pulse</u> your torso up and down; the movements should not be more than a couple inches up and down.

NOTE: make sure that <u>your shoulders never go lower than the "starting position"</u>, (which is where you lifted "comfortably high", as in the photo on the previous page). Your lower back should be constantly pressed to the floor, AND you Ab muscles should never relax; they should be constantly pulled into your body.

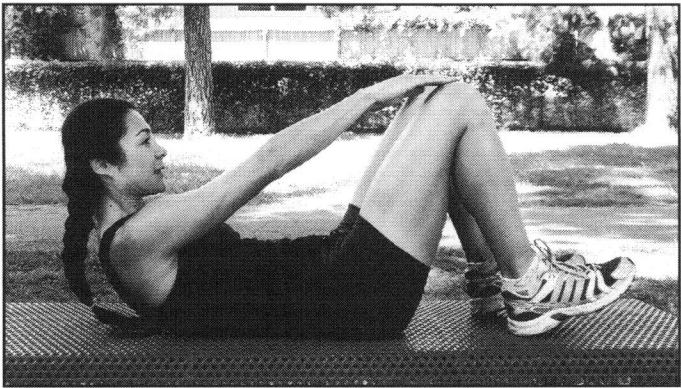

6. Move-up and down like this for 10 pulse repetitions.

7. Do 3 sets.

<u>Advancing</u>:
Add 5 repetitions at a time, until you are up to 25 repetitions per set.

Goal - Micro-Crunches TM:
1 time a day - 3 sets of 25 repetitions

Introduction: Toe-taps TM

Targeting "lower-abs", (below the belly button). Improve control and strength of your "lower abs", and entire core.

Toe-taps TM:

1. Lay on the floor, onto your back. Lift your feet and bring your thighs into your body. Lay your arms down next to the sides of your body.

(see photo on the next page)

Toe Taps TM

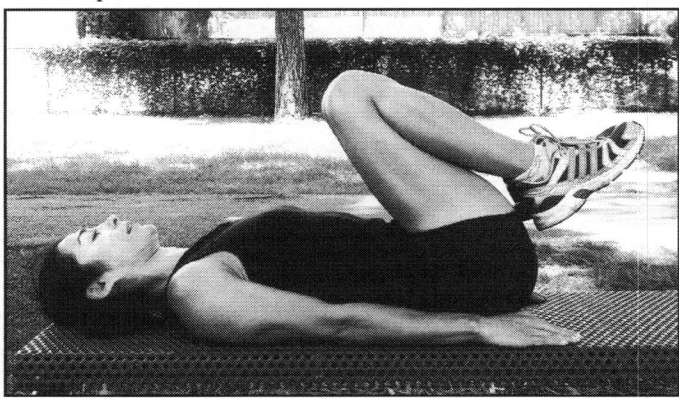

2. Press your lower back into the floor, and tightly pull-in your ab muscles.

3. While keeping your lower back CONTINUOUSLY pressed into the floor, and keeping your abs TIGHLTY pulled into your body, very slowly lower you feet to the floor until you lightly touch the floor with your toes. *Note: Keep your legs in the tucked position.*

Toe Taps TM – feet are in lower position

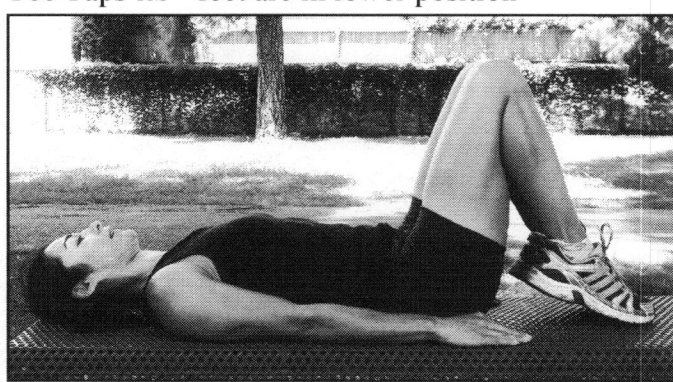

4. While keeping you lower back CONTINUOUSLY pressed into the floor, and abs TIGHLTY pulled into your body, slowly take your toes off the floor, and return your legs back to the starting position, (tucked into your body).

5. Do this under COMPLETE CONTROL, 3 times in a row.

Advancing:

Add one repetition at a time until you are up to 10 repetitions.

Important Note: Do not add repetitions until you are capable with doing however many you are already doing in complete control, (with your lower back pressed into the floor, AND ab muscles tightly pulled into your body, THROUGHOUT the entire movement.

Goal - Toe-Taps ᴛᴍ:
1 time a day - 2 sets of 10 repetitions

14ᵗʰ week – 17ᵗʰ week: *(remember to use the "check-off sheets" as reference)*
Once Daily – 2 sets of Micro-crunches ᴛᴍ, 2 sets of Toe Taps ᴛᴍ, 1 set of Half and Half Planks
ᴛᴍ

Almost There!
All you have left to add to your abdominal rehab program
are the Ishio Method - Abdominal Rehab Maintenance Exercises ᴛᴍ

It is critical for your continued improvements, and long-term maintenance, that you continue doing abdominal exercises. On page 54 is a complete maintenance protocol; follow the principles daily, and do the exercises a few times a week.

You can also add your favorite core exercises too

Ishio Method – Abdominal Rehab Maintenance Program ᴛᴍ

* Make habit, Ishio Method – Post Pregnancy Rehab Key Principles ᴛᴍ
*Continue wearing the Sillo Belly Wrap ᴛᴍ at night while you sleep, (crossing in back)

Three exercises: Off-Bench Crunches ᴛᴍ, Hip Lifts, and Regular Planks

(The next 3 exercises are simply more advanced versions of what you have already done so far)

Introducing: Off-Bench Crunches ™

Pulling the two halves of your "six-pack" together, flattening the stomach, making the abs even stronger.

Off-Bench Crunches ™:

1. Use a gym flat bench, park bench, or something very similar.

Note: If using a hard bench, fold a towel and lay it onto the bench as cushion for your mid and lower back.

2. Lay on the bench, onto your back.
3. Press your lower back into the bench, and tightly pull-in your ab muscles.
4. Now scoot back until your shoulder blades are off the bench, and re-check your lower back and ab positions.

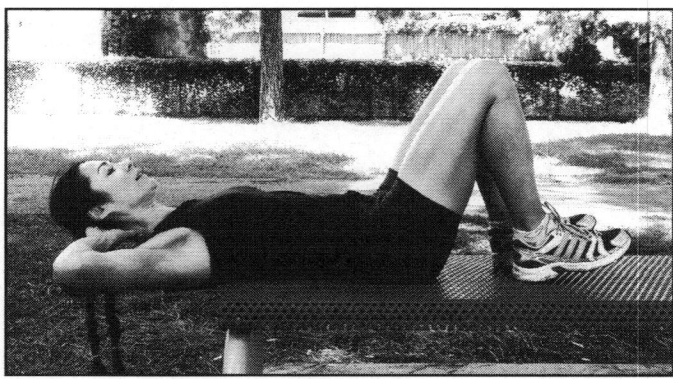

Note: you can do this with your arms crossed in front of your chest or with your hands behind your head. Having your hand behind you head is the harder version because the weight of your arms adds to the difficulty.

5. <u>Leading with your shoulders</u>, move up and down; you only need to go up and down about 3 inches. <u>ALWAYS keep your lower back pressed into the bench, and ALWAYS keep your Ab muscles "pulled-in" tightly</u>.

(see photo on the next page)

Off-Bench Crunches ™ – "up" position

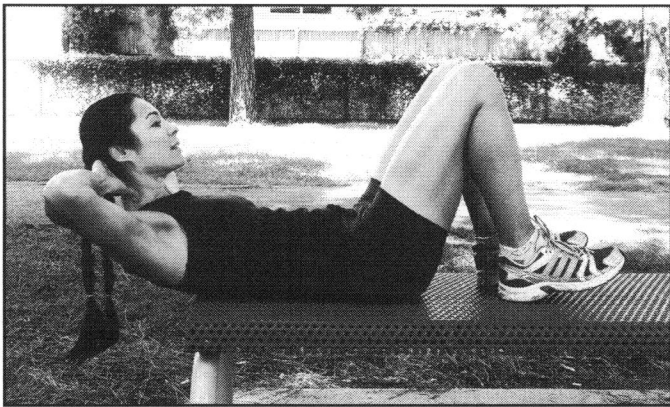

Note: If it is too hard to hold yourself up with your entire shoulder blades completely off the edge of the bench, then scoot in a little bit until you build up more strength; as you get stronger, slowly work more of your shoulder blades off the bench.

Advancing:
Increase in increments of 5 until you reach 25 repetitions.

Goal - Off-bench Crunches ™:
At least 3 times a week – 2 - 3 sets of 25 repetitions.
* If you do not have access to a bench, then **do Micro Crunches ™ instead** *

Introduction: Hip Lifts

Targeting "lower-abs", (below the belly button). Improve control and strength of your "lower abs", and entire core.

Hip Lifts:

1. Lay on the floor, onto your back. Lift your feet and bring your thighs into your body. Lay your arms down next to the sides of your body. This is your starting position.

(see photo on the next page)

Hip Lifts – Start Position

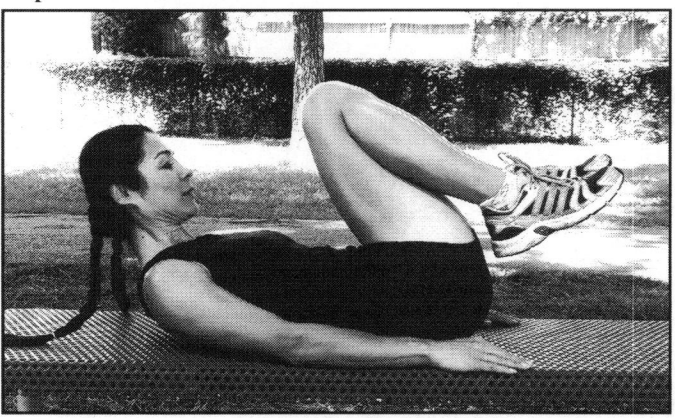

Note: You can either raise your head/shoulders slightly off the floor, or keep them completely flat on the floor. For most, it's easier when lifting the head/shoulders slightly off the floor.

2. Press your lower back into the floor, and TIGHLTY pull-in your Ab muscles.

3. Now lift your hips off the floor, (like you are curling them into your chest). To help with lifting your hips, you will want to press your palms into the floor, as you curl up.

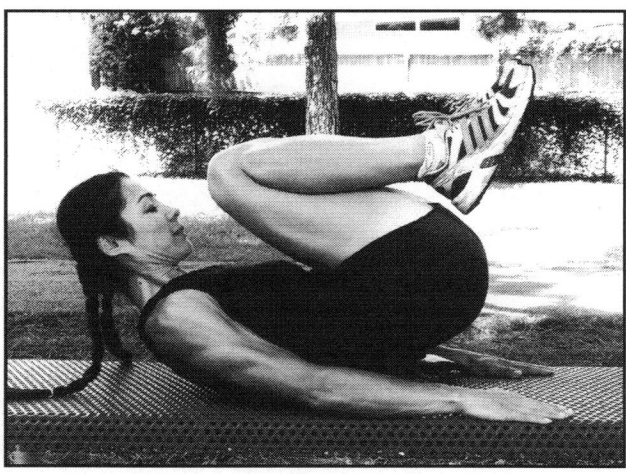

4. Come down SLOWLY, in complete CONTROL, the ENTIRE TIME…and repeat.

Important Note: Never let your lower back "pop-up" off the floor, or allow your abs to relax, even when you are back down in the "starting position" about to start another repetition; always stay tight and under control.

Advancing:
Increase repetitions of 1 or 2, until you reach 10 repetitions.

Goal - Hip Lifts:
At least 3 times a week - 2 sets of 10 repetitions.

Introduction: Regular Planks (on elbows)

Improve total core strength, including upper body strength, and posture.

Regular Planks (on elbows):

1. Kneel on the floor, onto your hands and knees.
2. Pull-in your abdominal muscles as tightly as you can.
3. Go down onto your forearms to hold up your body, and move your legs out one at a time, until they are both straight.
4. Re-check to make sure that your abdominal muscles are "pulled-in", that you have "good posture", (shoulders drawn back, chest opened), and your hips are not "drooping down".

Correct

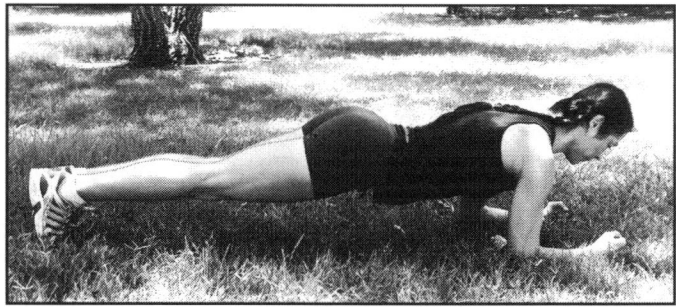

Incorrect

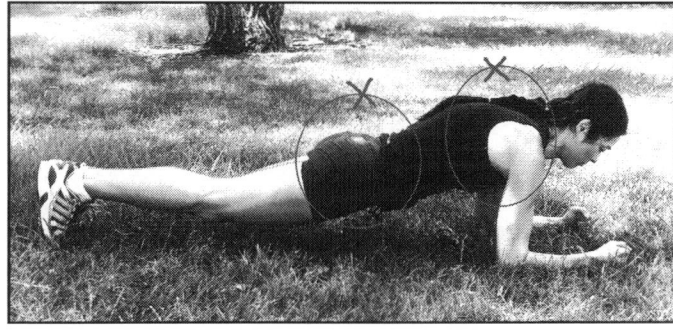

5. Hold for 20 seconds.

Advancing:
Start adding increments of 5 seconds, until you are at 45 - 60 seconds.

Goal - Regular Planks (on elbows):
At least 3 times a week - 2 sets of 45 -60 seconds.

Ishio Method - Abdominal Rehab Maintenance Protocol ™

Main Principles	**Set Posture ™ and Surge Posture ™**
• Core Posture ™ • Surge Posture ™ • Set Posture ™ • Breathe Posture ™	• While Exercising

---

Ab Circuit: (Do at least 3 times a week)

Regular Planks - 2 sets - 30 - 60 seconds per set.

Off-Bench Crunches ™ - 3 sets - 25 count
Do Micro-crunches ™ if you don't have access to a bench

Hip Lifts ™ - 2 sets of 10 count

Important Note: Quality versus Quantity

• During the exercises, keep your abdominal muscles "tight" at all times; don't relax them. The time to relax your abs are in between sets, (which are the designated rest times).

Reminders:

By maintaining proper Core Posture ™, and doing Surge Postures ™ throughout the day when doing "normal" activities, you will automatically be helping maximize the toning of your Ab muscles.

Through conscious Surge Posture ™ practice, eventually, whenever exerting yourself, your Ab muscles will have an "automatic reaction" of contracting "in", without having to think about it.

As your Ab muscles increase in density, you will require much less thoughts or efforts with maintaining Set Posture ™ throughout everyday living.

Chapter Five:

Nutritional Guidance

Postpartum Supportive Nutritional Guidance

We need supportive nutrition to help reduce inflammation, to heal, and balance back our hormones, (which can also help us avoid or lessen the severity of postpartum depression or postpartum anxiety).

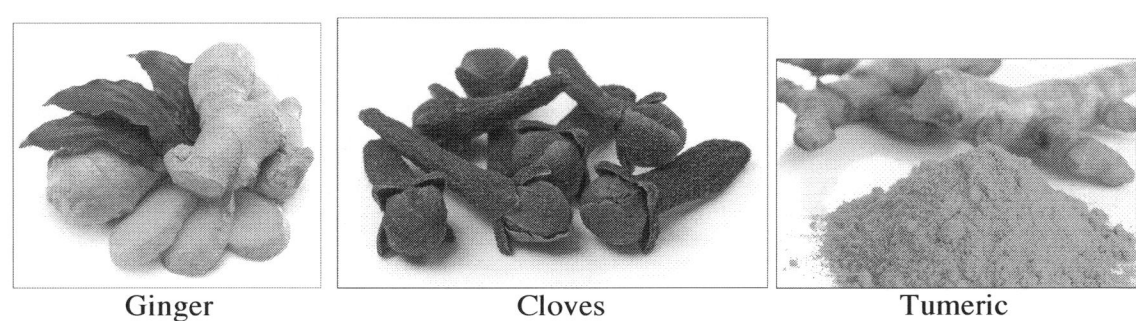

Ginger   Cloves   Tumeric

Right after delivering our baby, our body goes through a rapid major hormonal shift. We NEED proper nutrition to assist our body with smoothly transitioning through the hormones of pregnancy and delivery, to pre-pregnancy levels.

When we properly support our hormone changes with proper nutrition, we help lessen the severity, or avoid, baby blues, postpartum depression, stress induced anxiety, significant sleep disturbances, and of the like.

When we properly support our hormone changes with proper nutrition, we also support our body's physical repair process by help lessening inflammation. Good nutrition also helps purge the excess water weight that we gained.

HAVE LOT'S OF:

Omega-Fats – Our brain shrinks while we are pregnant, and adding omega fats can help "plump it back up". Omegas are also anti-inflammatories, and they have been known to regulate some hormones. *Examples: Omega supplements, seafood, flax, wild rice, walnuts, pasteurized raised meats, omega enriched diary foods, and omega enriched eggs.*

Fluids – This includes water, AND broths (soups). Your body's average pH level is about 7.5, and water helps balance your pH levels from foods you eat that raise it, (i.e. sugars); hence, water helps as an anti-inflammatory. Broths have lots of nutrients in it also, so it's supportive of your body's healing, (and as a bonus, broth soups are very soothing).

Green Vegetables – such as spinach; help restore the body's proper pH.

Eat Organic – whenever possible, ESPECIALLY the first 3 months after having your baby. If 3 months is out of your budget, then prioritize your first 6-weeks. Most of the fruits and vegetables we eat today have been grown/sprayed with chemicals, and these chemicals affects our hormones, and inflammation in our body.

If budget is a significant issue, then buy organic for the foods that you don't peel or that have thin skin, (i.e. apples, grapes, lettuce), and buy non-organic for the foods you do peel, (i.e. banana's, oranges). Since you are a recovering mom, it's OK if it means that these organic food are set-aside just for you to eat during this first 6-12 weeks postpartum; the entire family can be on-board for someone who is always caring for them ☺.

Eat Meats and Dairy That Are Grass Fed and Free Range - whenever possible, ESPECIALLY the first 3 months after having your baby. If 3 months is out of your budget, then prioritize your first 6-weeks.

Grass fed/free range meats offer many fatty acids missing in the Standard American Diet, in contrary, grain fed animals have too much omega-6's, and not enough omega-3's, (such as corn). All this affects our hormones, and inflammation in our body.

LIMIT:

Too Much Omega-6 Fats – although they compliment Omega-3 Fats, they also promote inflammation, so you want to make sure you don't have too much, (at least during the immediate 6-12 weeks postpartum phase). *Examples are corn, and edamame.*

Refined Sugars - Sugar offers insignificant amounts of vitamins and minerals, and is an inflammatory in our bodies. Avoid too much sugary snacks, and even high glycemic vegetables, and fruits while recovering from having a baby.

TOP 3 favorite anti-inflammatory foods:
(chosen by nutritionists are)

Ginger

What is it? Ginger is the underground rhizome of the ginger plant, also known botanically as Zingiber officinale. Ginger is aromatic, pungent, and spicy.
Why does it work? Ginger contains very potent anti-inflammatory compounds called gingerols.
How can I use it? *Add ginger to your drinks: homemade lemonade, and teas. *Add it to your Asian rice dishes by sprinkling grated ginger on top. *Add ginger to an olive oil and garlic based salad dressing.

Cloves

What is it? Cloves are the unopened pink flower buds of the evergreen clove tree. Cloves are warm, sweet, and have an aromatic taste.
Why does it work? The primary component of clove's volatile oils called Eugenol functions as an anti-inflammatory substance.
How can I use it? Cloves have a very intense flavor, especially when they have been ground, so it is always better to go light when adding them to your recipes'. *Peirce an onion with cloves, and add it to soups, and broths. *Add cloves, and cinnamon, to warm apple cider, or teas. *

Tumeric

What is it? Turmeric comes from the root of the Curcuma Longa plant. Turmeric has a warm, peppery, and bitter flavor. Its fragrance has a hint of orange, and ginger.
Why does it work? Tumeric's volatile oil has significant anti-inflammatory activity. Even more potent than its volatile oil is the yellow or orange pigment, which is called Curcumin. Curcumin's anti-inflammatory effects have been shown to be comparable to the western drugs such as hydrocortisone, and over-the-counter anti-inflammatory medicines.
How can I use it? *Add to curry of course, since that is one of the main ingredients to prepare curry. *Sprinkle turmeric over eggs. *Sprinkle over steamed vegetables, (cauliflower, green beans, onions). *Add to salad dressing.

Nutrition Plan General Guideline

Important Note: This is only intended as a guideline. If you have any special dietary restriction or needs, that particular nutritional protocol needs to super seed any information contained in this book.

This "Nutrition Plan General Guideline" **IS**:

* Simplified explanations of some nutrition basics.
* "Friendly" towards making realistic nutritional lifestyle changes.
* Adaptable: allowing you to create a more personalized plan of healthier eating that can be based off of your own personal food preferences, (i.e. likes, dislikes, cultural, religious).
* Flexible with your personal daily time schedule.

This "Nutrition Plan General Guideline" **IS NOT**:

* Very restrictive: only allowing you to eat certain things, or at certain times.
* A precise plan, specific to any health circumstance.

Important Tools Available to Help With Success: (sheet are in chapter 12)

Lifestyle Log: this is especially important for those that have poor nutritional habits, (food choices, over-eating, under-eating, or having long periods go by without eating).

The Lifestyle Log is so you can get an idea of what your current nutritional, (and exercise), habits are. Log for 1 full week, review at the end of that week, and you will be able to see your habits accurately. Make notes on any necessary adjustments you need to make, while continue logging for at least another few months, (and longer if needed to maintain discipline).

After using the Lifestyle Log for a little while, eventually, you will be able to simply reflect on your day/week and know if you are still "in" the nutritional and exercise plan that is part of your personal health "zone".

Top Ten Food Favorites Sheet: this is a reference sheet for a quick way to recall your favorite foods and portion sizes that is based off your needs. By filling it out in the first place, it helps you reinforce at a conscious and subconscious level, what your plan is.

Nutrition Plan - 6 Principles

It should be noted that most of the principles tie into each other with the same concept.

#1: Portion control is key.

Fill-out the "Caloric Needs Estimator" sheet that is included later in this chapter, (on pages 63 and 64). <u>It is important that you stay within the range that is figured by the worksheet.</u>

#2: Don't under eat.

Your body needs fuel to maintain it's normal functioning, (i.e. keep your heart beating, breathing, skin repairing, muscle maintenance, etc.). Your body also needs calories to sustain normal activity, (i.e. walking, house cleaning, taking a shower, etc). Lastly, you body needs fuel to sustain formal exercising..

If you don't give your body the fuel it needs, it will take the nutrients/energy it needs from your muscles.

Whenever you are hungry, don't think to yourself that you are burning body fat, and understand that you are burning your precious muscles. Prioritize eating something, even if just to hold you over until you can properly eat within the next hour.

#3: Eat within 1 hour of waking up.

It doesn't matter if you have a sit down breakfast, or eat something quickly to hold you over for an additional hour until you can have a "real" meal.

Many people have said, "But I'm not hungry for breakfast", and often my reply is, "You have trained your body to not be hungry for long periods at a time". If you don't eat until many hours after waking up, or go for long periods throughout the day without eating, you are training your body to slow down its metabolism.

Since you are going to have a long busy day, you need to jumpstart your system, and give it what it needs to get it going. Also eating nutritious foods will limit mood swings, and maintain sustained energy.

#4: Don't let more than 4 hours go by without eating something.

If you don't eat throughout the day, you will affect your hormones; not just metabolism, but you are also affecting your mood, and energy.

Many of my clients have said, "won't I be burning fat", and the simple answer is, you will not be "burning fat", you will be "burning muscle".

#5: Usually, don't eat within 2 hours of going to bed.

If you notice here, I did not say, "do not eat after 8.m." or "6p.m", or etc. Many people have voiced their confusion and concern regarding the rigid times noted.

Everyone has a different life schedule, work schedule, etc, so you can't put a definitive time on what time you are not allowed to eat past. If you work until 1am, it's unhealthy if you were not to eat past 6pm or 8pm; your body needs fuel since you will still be up, moving around, and working.

I also noted "usually" for a reason. If your stomach is growling, and even though it's within 2 hours of going to bed, you need to eat something since your body is definitely telling you it needs food. Eat something "light" and "small", keeping the snack high in lean protein, and low in complex carbohydrates/sugars, (i.e. chicken and vegetables).

#6: Eat green everyday.

In the average U.S. diet, we usually don't have a problem with getting in carbohydrates and proteins; what we have shown is our lack of vegetables and fruits intake.

The "Centers for Disease Control and Prevention" (CDC) keeps it very clear by telling you how many cups you need daily. http://www.fruitsandveggiesmatter.gov/index.html

In this chapter, it also lists how much vegetables, fruits, meats/beans, grains, and dairy you need daily, (based off of your "daily caloric needs").

Reduce Body Fat

If you have been over-eating, then you need to cut those extra calories immediately. Make sure you complete the BMR "Caloric Needs Estimate" in Step 1, and then use the "Lifestyle Log" for a week to figure out your accurate current eating habits. Now, compare the difference in calories between your BMR "Caloric Needs Estimate", and your actual daily caloric intake; any difference needs to be cut immediately.

If you have sizeable enough body fat to lose, you can cut a few calories from your BMR - "Caloric Needs Estimate" from Step 1, (to add with the caloric deficit you are creating with your exercising). For many people, don't cut more than 200 calories per day from the estimate amount, <u>and</u> keep in mind, this is only supposed to be temporary. You don't want to cut too many calories, or else you can lose muscle density; you also run the high risk of mood and energy swings.

Stay within your appropriate calorie/nutrition range AND use exercise as the main means for creating a caloric deficit towards losing fat/weight. Exercising will also help keep you from losing lean body mass, (muscle), if cutting nutrition calories to create an extra temporary caloric deficit. <u>Exercise WILL keep you fit, manage moods, create a nicer physique, and build your confidence as your body goes through the weight loss transition</u>. If you are already exercising, then depending on what you are already doing, you may need to increase your exercise intensity, days, duration, and/or form of exercises.

Don't forget to re-calculate your "Caloric Needs Estimate" periodically. As your weight goes down, your caloric needs go down. As well, once you reach your goal weight/body fat, remember to add the "Caloric Needs Estimate Step 2" to the "Step 1" number, so you can properly maintain your weight/physique.

When you are maintaining your goal weight/physique, re-calculate your "Caloric Needs Estimate" if your activity level goes up, since then your caloric needs goes up, (i.e. training for a 5K).

Good news! **Once you are down to your goal weight/physique, and you are in the "Maintenance Mode", you will use the calories burned from exercising, as calories you get to consume. It's with these calories that makes "maintaining" more flexible and fun.**

(this area is left blank intentionally, continue reading on next page)

Caloric Needs Estimate - Step 1 of 2

BMR Formula (Basal Metabolic Rate)
The amount of calories your body needs to sustain "normal" bodily functioning, and activities, (such as walking, etc).

Do these calculations first:

A: 4.35 X your weight in pounds = _____.
B: 4.7 X your height in inches = _____.
C: 4.7 X your age in years = _____.

 # 1: Add "A" and "B" together, then add it to 655 = _____.

 # 2: Subtract "C" from the answer from "# 1" = _____.

The answer from Step #2 is your personal BMR.

EXAMPLE:

30 year old
5'4" (64 inches)
140 pounds

BMR Formula (in pounds)

Do these calculations first:

A: 4.35 X (140 pounds) = 609
B: 4.7 X (64 inches) = 300.8
C: 4.7 X your age in years = 141

 # 1: Add "A" and "B" together, then add it to 655 = 1564.8
(609 + 300.8 + 655 = 1564.8)

 # 2: Subtract "C" from the answer from "# 1" = **1,424 calories (rounded up)**
(1564.8 - 141 = 1,423.8 calories)

GO TO THE "STEP 2" FINISH YOUR CALORIC NEEDS ESTIMATE

63

Important: <u>Step 2 is for once you reach your goal weight/body fat level</u>, and you are in "maintenance mode". <u>When you are trying to cut weight/fat, you don't add the calories from Step 2 into your "daily caloric needs estimate"</u>; you will use the exercise calories burned, as the main caloric deficit you create towards cutting your excess fat/weight.

Caloric Needs Estimate - <u>Step 2 of 2</u>

Harris Benedict Formula

Multiply your BMR (Step 1 you just completed) with an activity factor below.

Sedentary: little or no exercise: Your BMR X 1.2

Lightly Active: light exercise/sports 1-3 days a week: Your BMR X 1.375

Moderately Active: moderate exercise/sports 3-5 days a week: Your BMR X 1.55

Very Active: hard exercise/sports 6-7 days a week" Your BMR X 1.725

Extra Active: very hard exercise/sports & physical job or 2X training: Your BMR X 1.9

Your BMR multiplied by an exercise factor = <u>Your Total Daily Caloric Needs</u>

(Activity level number) _____ X (BMR from step 1) _____ = _____

EXAMPLE:

30 year old
5'4" (64 inches)
140 pounds
Lightly Active

Multiply your BMR (Step 1 you just completed) with an activity factor below.

(Lightly Active) <u>1.375</u> X (BMR from step 1) <u>1,424</u> = 1958 calories a day to maintain weight.

Common Food Ratio Goal

15% Protein
25% Fat - not more than 10% as saturated fat, (i.e. butter)
60% Carbohydrates

* For people that have special needs for health concerns, or athletic needs, please consult a nutritionist, or an expert in that particular field. *

U.S. Government Dietary Guidelines: 2010

Recommendation for 1400 calorie-a-day
Fruits - 1 ½ cups
Vegetables - 1 ½ cups
Meat and Beans - 4 ounces
Grains - 5 ounces (2 ½ ounces should be whole grains such as multi-grain bread)
Dairy - 2 cups

Recommendation for 1600 calorie-a-day
Fruits - 1 ½ cups
Vegetables - 2 cups
Meat and Beans - 5 ounces
Grains - 5 ounces (½ should be whole grains such as multi-grain bread)
Dairy - 3 cups

Recommendation for 1800 calorie-a-day
Fruits - 1 ½ cups
Vegetables - 2 ½ cups
Meat and Beans - 5 ounces
Grains - 6 ounces (½ should be whole grains such as multi-grain bread)
Dairy - 3 cups

Recommendation for 2000 calorie-a-day

Fruits - 2 cups

Vegetables - 2 ½ cups

Meat and Beans - 5 ½ ounces

Grains - 6 ounces (½ should be whole grains such as multi-grain bread)

Dairy - 3 cups

Recommendation for 2200 calorie-a-day

Fruits - 2 cups

Vegetables - 3 cups

Meat and Beans - 6 ounces

Grains - 7 ounces (½ should be whole grains such as multi-grain bread)

Dairy - 3 cups

Recommendation for 2400 calorie-a-day

Fruits - 2 cups

Vegetables - 3 cups

Meat and Beans - 6 ½ ounces

Grains - 8 ounces (½ should be whole grains such as multi-grain bread)

Dairy - 3 cups

Recommendation for 2600 calorie-a-day

Fruits - 2 cups

Vegetables - 3 ½ cups

Meat and Beans - 6 ½ ounces

Grains - 9 ounces (½ should be whole grains such as multi-grain bread)

Dairy - 3 cups

Portion List

Please Note: This next section is a close estimate only, please read your food labels, and cooking method for more accurate calorie counts.

Fruit

1 cup = 1 large banana (approx: 121 calories)
1 cup = 8 large strawberries (approx: 48 calories)
1 cup = 15 grapes (approx: 51 calories)
1 cup = 2 large plums (approx: 61 calories)
1 cup = 1 apple (approx: 95 calories)
1 cup = 1 pear (approx: 103 calories)

Vegetable

1 cup = 1 cup cooked vegetables (approx: 110 calories)
1 cup = 2 cups of raw leafy greens (approx: 10 calories)
1 cup = 1 large ear of corn (approx: 127 calories)
1 cup = 10 broccoli florets (approx: 52 calories)
1 cup = 12 baby carrots (approx: 42 calories)

Lean meat

4 ounces = 1 medium size chicken breast, broiled or fired, meat only (approx: 212 calories)
4 ounces = 2 medium chicken thighs, broiled or fried, meat only (approx: 247 calories)
4 ounces = 2 ½ medium chicken legs, broiled or fried, meat only (approx: 236 calories)
4 ounces = 4 slices of turkey meat (approx: 112 calories)
4 ounces = salmon (approx: 234 calories)
4 ounces = white fish (approx: 195 calories)

Other proteins

1 large egg = (approx: 90 calories)
1 ounce = mixed nuts with salt = (approx: 168 calories)
4 ounces = ½ cup Snap Beans (approx: 26 calories)
4 ounces = ½ cup Pinto Beans (approx: 22 calories)
4 ounces = ½ cup Kidney Beans (approx: 37 calories)
4 ounces = ½ cup Lima Beans (approx: 80 calories)

Grains

2 ounces = 2 slices of regular multi-grain bread (approx: 138 calories)
5 ounces = little more than ¾ cup of brown rice (approx: 158 calories)
5 ounces = little more than ¾ cup of white rice (approx: 184 calories)
5 ounces = little more than ¾ cup of oatmeal (approx: 132 calories)

Dairy

1 cup 1% Milk (approx: 102 calories)
1 cup 2% Milk (approx: 122 calories)
½ cup = shredded cheddar cheese (approx: 177 calories)
1 cup = cottage cheese 1% (approx: 163 calories)
1 cup = yogurt light with fruit (approx: 100 calories)

(this area is left blank intentionally, continue reading on next page)

Nutrition Plan Example

1400-calorie meal plan (following the U.S. Government Dietary Guideline 2010)

Note: If you are on a higher calorie plan, then simply add the extra calories/nutrition recommendations to this nutrition plan. Also, this is a close estimate only, please read your food labels, and cooking method for more accurate calorie/nutrition counts.

Wake-up: 6:45am

Jumpstart: 7am
* 1 cup water, and ½ large banana (60 calories / ½ cup fruit)

First meal: 8am
* 1 cup oatmeal with ½ peach, and 1 teaspoon of honey. (180 calories / 6 ounces of grain / ½ cup fruit)

Snack: 10am
* Protein shake with 1% milk (250 calories / 1 cup dairy / ½ cup fruit/ 25 grams of protein)

Second meal: noon
* Turkey sandwich (2 slices of whole wheat bread, mustard, salt/pepper, tomato, lettuce, 4 slices of sandwich turkey meat) (320 calories / 2 ounces grain / 2 ounces meat / 1 cup vegetables)
* Large plum (30 calories / ½ cup fruit)

Snack: 4pm
* Light yogurt (any flavor) (90 calories / 1 cup dairy)

Third meal: 6:30pm
* 1 pieces of chicken (thigh, no skin) (123 calories / 2 ounces of meat)
* Rice - 1/2 cup (100 calories / 3.25 ounces of grain)
* Broccoli – 2 cups (100 calories / 1 ½ cups vegetable)
* Real chocolate ice cream ½ cup (147 calories / ½ cup dairy)

Bedtime: 10:45pm

Totals: <u>1400 calories.</u>
Servings: <u>Fruits</u> – 2 cups, <u>Vegetables</u> – 2.5 cups, <u>Meat/Beans</u> - 4 ounces, <u>Grains</u> – 11.25, (8 ounces of it is high in fiber), and <u>Dairy</u> – 2.5 cups, <u>Protein supplement</u> - 25 grams of whey protein to support weight lifting/training, <u>Calcium supplement</u>, and <u>Multi-vitamin</u>.

Golden Rule for Moms

"I AM as IMPORTANT as my children".
Do for ourselves as we do for our children.
It doesn't have to equal the same amount of time,
but it has to equal the same amount of care.

Awareness that you have the ability and responsibility to design the ambiance of your life is powerful wisdom to have; its creativity and productivity are endless.

Chapter Six:

Balansu Therapy ™
re-adjust posture, relieve pain, rejuvenate body

Lower Backache

Improve your posture (standing)

Stand with the "Ideal Core Box Posture". (As was already discussed on page 15 & 16)

Some reminder directions on next page…

(overly "sticking out")   (ideal position)   (overly "tucked under")

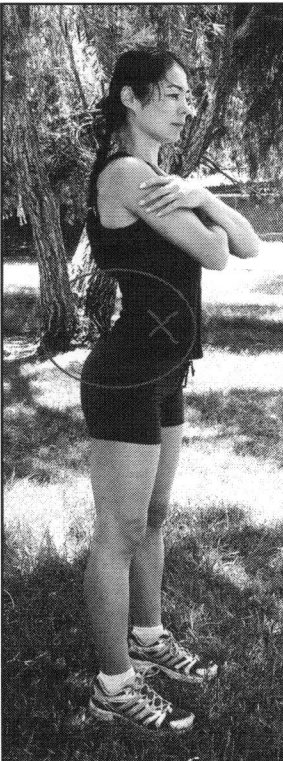 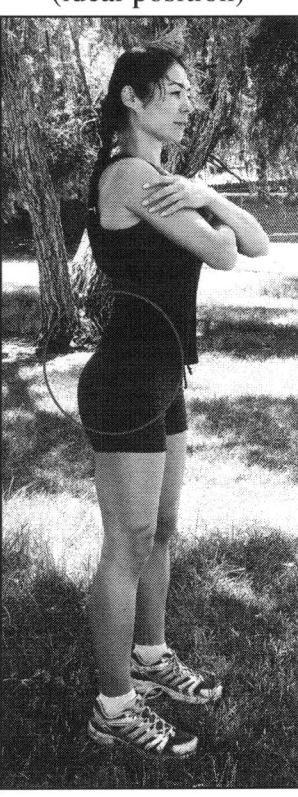 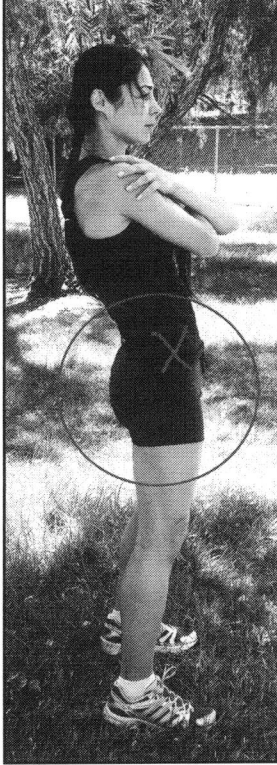

Getting into the Ideal Core Box Posture ™: The easiest way for most people to acquaint themselves with how to do this is, to start by standing side-ways next to a mirror. Now imagine that there is a medium size circle stuck to the side of your hip, and a vertical line sticking out of the top of the circle. Start by "overly sticking your butt out backwards", (like the photo above on the right), and now slowly rotate your pelvis around counter clockwise, (which means the line at the top of the circle will turn counter clockwise). When looking in the mirror side-ways as you do this, you should see your belly button area contract in towards your body, WHILE you lower back lengthens/straightens out a bit. *Be sure not to simply push your pelvis area forward incorrectly, (like the photo on the previous page).*

Keep practicing if you don't get it the first time, most people take many tries.

A reference example: think back to when wearing high-heeled shoes for a night out, and by the middle/end of the night, your lower back being achy? When wearing high-heeled shoes, it changes your posture automatically to "overly arching" your lower back, and "lifting your tailbone"; doing this puts extra pressure on your lower back, (as with the very left photo). Next time when wearing high-heeled shoes, give your lower back a break by going into the "Ideal Core Box Posture", and you will see it makes a huge difference on instantly taking the lower back pain away.

Improve your posture (when leaning forward)

This section is especially important after having a baby because the lower back usually gets painful when leaning forward and/or lifting things, (i.e. changing the baby's diaper).

Note: The back becomes very painful when leaning forward because after having a baby, our abdominal muscles are all stretched out and weak. When leaning forward, our body relies on our entire core for support and structure. When our abdominal muscles aren't strong enough to contribute properly, our back ends up doing most of the work. Also, when our muscles in general our weak, our body will start relying on our bones/tendons/ligaments to have to take on the extra load that the muscles aren't properly contributing to.

1. Before leaning forward, stick out you butt backwards AS you bend your knees AND straighten your entire back WHILE pulling in your abdominal muscles. This position will help distribute any pressure/weight throughout more of your body. In addition, it helps strengthen your abdominal muscles in the correct position.

(see photo on next page)

Correct　　　　　　　　　**Incorrect** – Don't have your lower back curled over

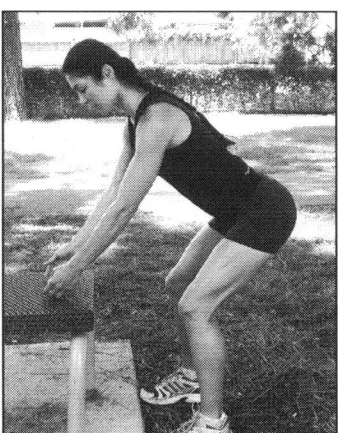 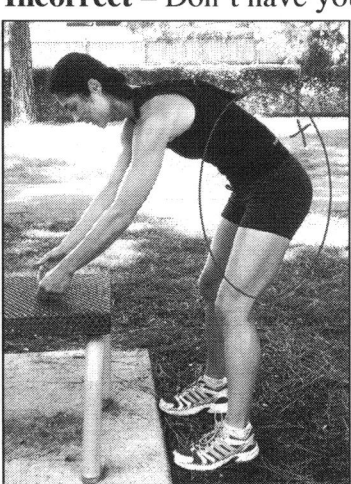

Strength training for lower back:

<u>While pregnant or shortly after delivery</u>

Do **Cat Backs**:
(This can also be used as a stretch).

1. Get on your hands and knees. Use a mat or towels for your knees. Gently "bend" your stomach towards the floor.

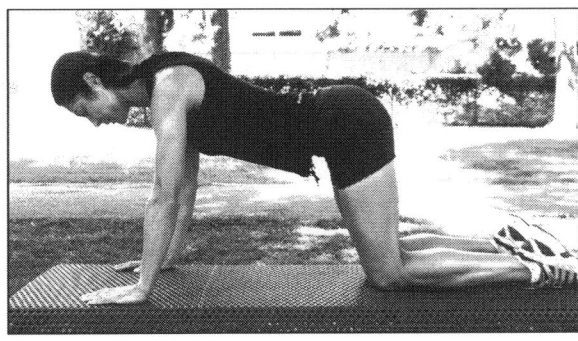

2. Next, curl your lower back up towards the ceiling.

(see photos on the next page)

73

Cat Back - Correct

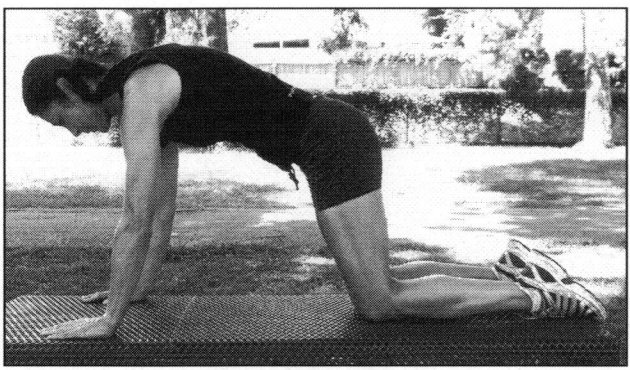

Cat Backs - Incorrect – Don't shrug your shoulders towards your ears.

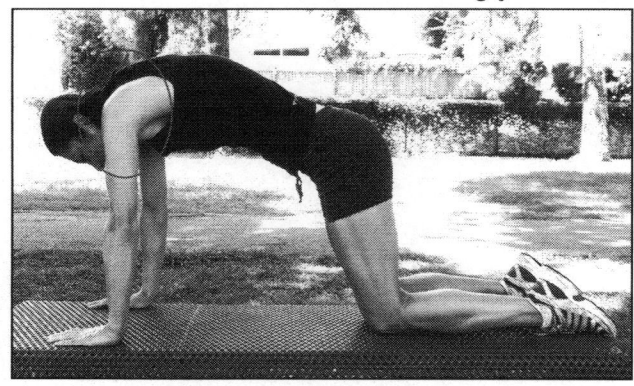

Keep your shoulders drawn back and down, as you curl your back up towards the ceiling; basically don't shrug your shoulders towards your ears. We want to stretch, strengthen, and relax; not add tension.

3. Slowly release back to the starting position, and repeat.

Do about 10 repetitions.

---

8 - 12-weeks after delivery
(consult your doctor before starting Super-mans if you had a C-section or have wide diastasis recti)

Do **Super-mans**:

Important: *While doing Super-mans, be sure not to "shrug" your shoulders, and keep your chest opened, (as with the "Planks" in the Ishio Method ᴛᴍ – Ab Rehab Program).*

Beginner level:

1. Lay on the floor with your belly side down.

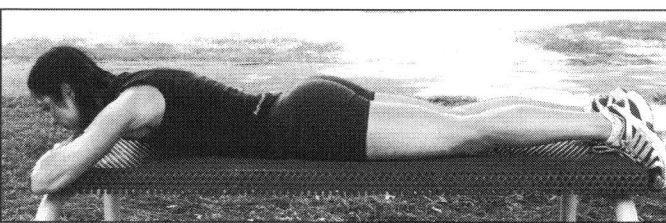

2. Tuck your hands under your chin with elbows out to the side.
3. Lift your torso off the ground for as long as you can, up to 20 seconds.

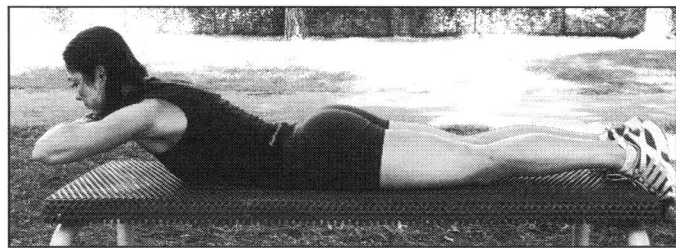

Do 3 sets.

Advancing: Once you can hold this position for 3 sets of 20 seconds, you are ready to go onto the "intermediate level".

Intermediate level:

1. Lay on the floor with your belly side down.
2. Straighten out your arms to the sides of your body.
3. Lift your torso and legs off the ground for as long as you can, up to 20 seconds.

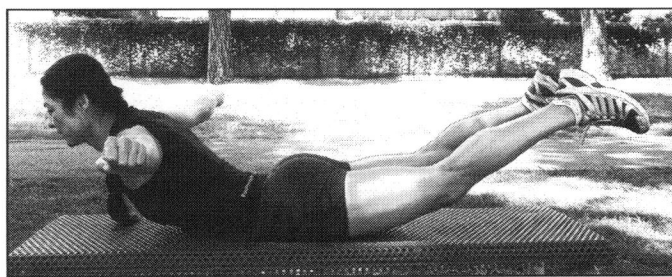

Do 3 sets.

Advancing: Once you can hold this "intermediate position" for 3 sets of 20 seconds, you are ready to go onto the "advanced level".

Advanced level:

1. Lay on the floor with your belly side down.
2. Straighten out your arms, straight ahead, in front of you.

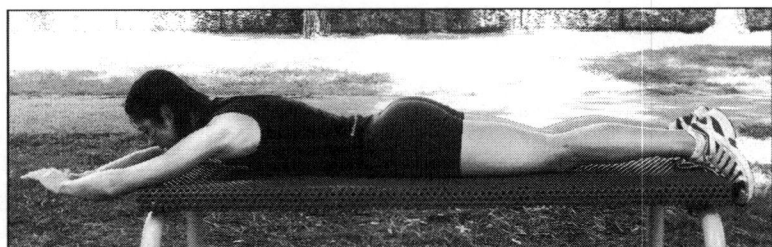

3. Lift your torso and legs off the ground for as long as you can, up to 30 seconds. <u>If you want it tougher, only lift your torso off the ground, and leave your legs on the ground the entire time.</u>

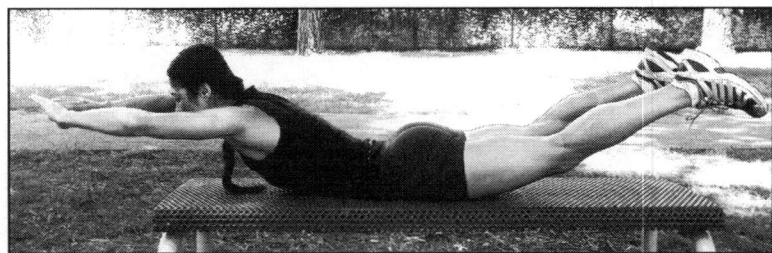

Do 3 sets

Do **Planks**:

<u>Many weeks after delivery</u> -
(consult your doctor before starting if you had a C-section)

Planks are part of the Ishio Method – Abdominal Rehab Protocol ™. I am recommending it again here because "Planks" help strengthen the entire core region, which helps alleviate back discomfort/pain.

Refer Back to chapter 3 if you need a reminder, for details and photos, on how to do Planks.

Very Important: <u>Start with the Incline Planks ™, then Half and Half Planks ™, and lastly Regular Planks, as required in the Ishio Method ™ – Ab Rehab Protocol ™. Do not skip the</u>

<u>order of progression</u> because it's important to build proper strength and form before moving onto more advanced levels.

Stretches for your lower back:

Do **Hamstring Stretch Position 1 (hips pushed forward)**

Note #1: it may seem strange that you are stretching your hamstring (back of leg), and it is under the section "stretches for your lower back"; it has been proven that if you have tight hamstrings, it often times contributes to lower back pain.

Note #2: if you are very tight, doing this particular hamstring stretch position will initially have you feel the stretch more in the back of your leg, than your lower back; but as your hamstrings get more flexible, you will feel the stretch equally in your lower back, (if not mostly there). *FYI: by keeping the stretching apparatus height not too high for your current flexibility level, you can still get a good lower back stretch, even if you are pretty tight.*

1. You will use a chair, sofa end, bench, etc., as your stretching apparatus.

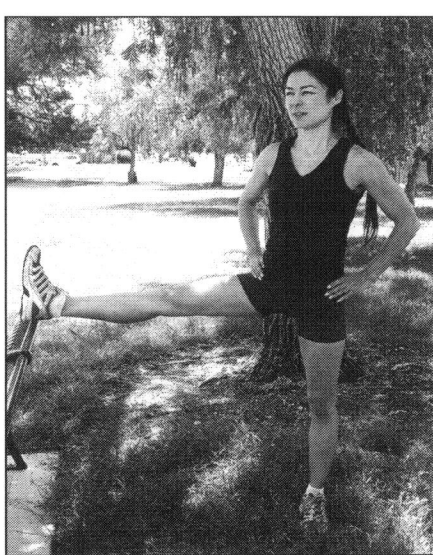

Important: How you decide on what "stretching apparatus" you need to use will be dependent on you current flexibility. A good place to start is a place that is a lower than you hip height; you can adjust higher as you become more flexible. When trying out a certain height, you should only feel a gentle pull in your hamstring, (back of your leg), and it should not be painful or force you into standing with bad posture, (i.e. hunching over when trying to straighten your leg).

2. Lift one foot up onto the object you chose as your "stretching apparatus". (See photo on previous page)

Notice: You want to have the back heel part of your shoe lying on the "stretching apparatus". Be sure not to irritate your Achilles tendon, (the tendon on the back of your foot, above the heel), by having that part lay on the "stretching apparatus".

3. With your "standing leg", (the leg on the floor), make sure your foot is **parallel**, (turned out), to the object you are standing in front of. *(see photo on previous page)*

4. Now, <u>push you hips forward</u>. This is an important detail to this stretch, since it will help take the stretch to your lower back. *(see front view photo, below)*

5. Take your "back arm", (the arm that is on the same side as your "standing leg"), and take it over your head, behind you, as you stretch your arm forward at the same time.

Front view   **Side View**

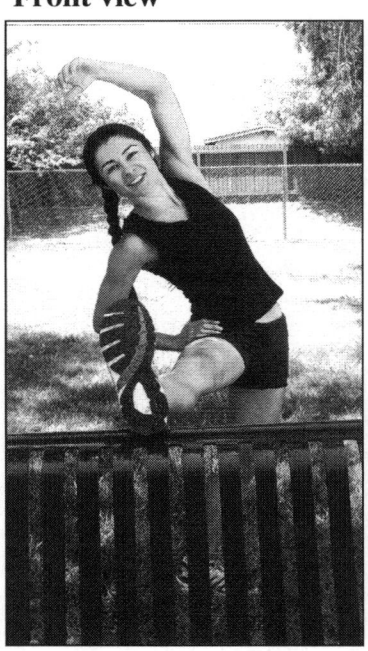 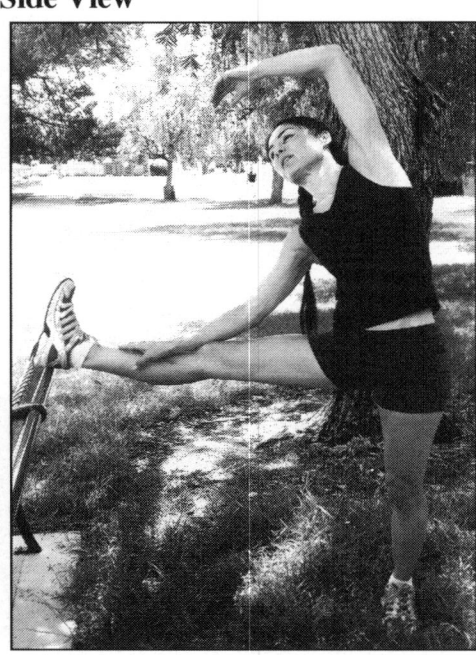

Important Note: Make sure that while you are taking your arm over your head, you are stretching it UP and OVER, to maximize the lower back stretch.

Notice: If you feel that you are off balance, make sure you have chair next to you so you can hold onto it if needed. If pregnant, you should always have a chair next to you for balance at all times.

****

Upper Backache

Improve your posture

Common "Bad" Posture:
Shoulders curled forward, with the chin protruding forward.

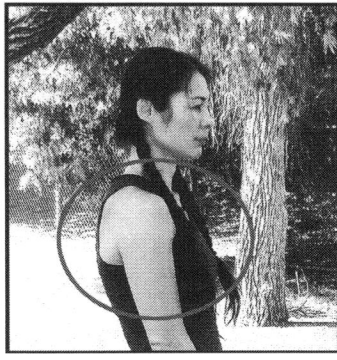

"Better" Posture:
Have your shoulders pulled Back AND Down.

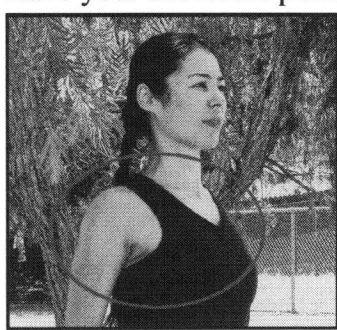

Strength training for your upper back:

Do **Seated Dumbbell Fly**. *(see photos on next page)*

1. Sit in a chair.
2. Move your butt closer to the edge of the chair and sit up tall, (shoulders back and down, chest opened, and abs pulled-in).
3. Take the heels of your feet off the floor so that you are on the balls of your feet.
4. While keeping your body tall, lean forward as far as possible without losing the tall posture, (don't "hunch" forward).
5. Start with both dumbbells down towards the ground.

6. Keeping your arms totally straight, (to make sure you are isolating your upper back as much as possible), lift the dumbbells out to the side.

Important Note: While lifting the dumbbells, <u>make sure</u> you are opening up your chest, and drawing your shoulder blades back as far as possible. This will help make sure you <u>don't collapse your body</u>, and you are actually using your upper back to lift the dumbbells.

7. Hold the dumbbells in the "up" position for half a second, then with complete control, lower the dumbbells down to the sides again.

Important Note: once your weights are at the bottom, <u>don't relax</u> your arms, keep them tight; in fact, don't "relax" your arms/upper back at any time during the set.

Do 2 - 3 sets of 8 – 15 repetitions, (and start with 3 – 5lbs)

Correct – shoulders drawn back, chest is opened up as you lift.

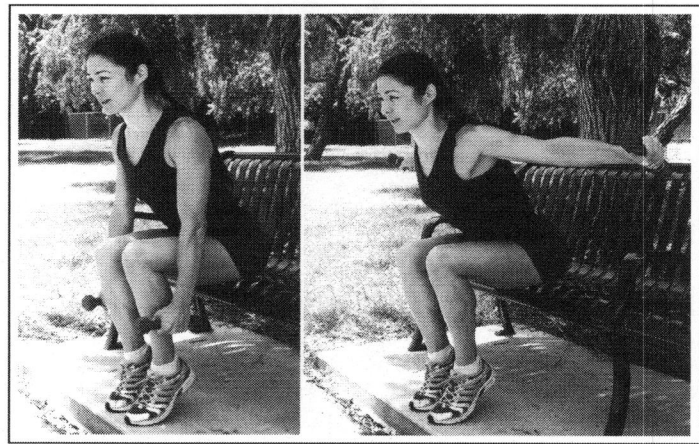

Incorrect – upper body collapsed, chest doesn't open.

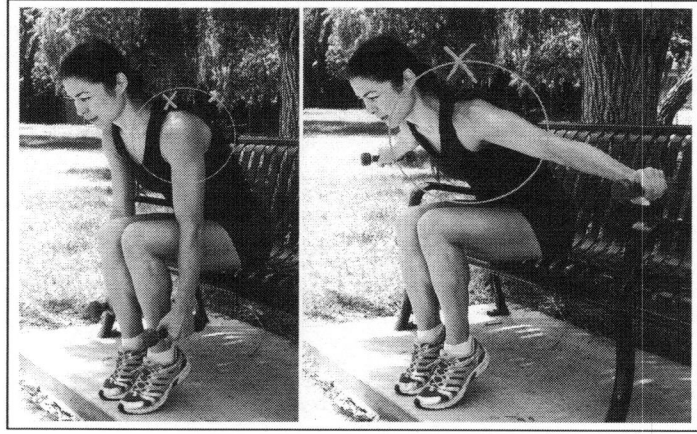

Stretches for your upper back

Do **Chest Stretch**:

Note: It may seem strange that you are stretching your chest, and it is under the section "stretches for your upper back". Often times, your upper back pain can be helped with better posture, and when you have tight chest muscles, it pulls your shoulders forward, causing you to have "bad" curved upper back posture. For "better" posture, it is just as important to have flexible chest muscles, as it is to have strong upper back muscles, so they are not constantly "fighting" each other.

By strengthening your upper back, while you stretch your chest, you will create a more balanced muscle state for your posture.

1. Stand at arms length away next to a fixed area such as a wall, a tree, or etc.
2. Gently close you hands into a fist and place on the side of the wall. The reason for the fist is to keep the entire arm relaxed, (and when not grabbing onto something, it helps with relaxing the arm). **Note:** your arm should be at about a 90-degree angle to your body. *(see photos below)*

3. Now, use your arm and push against the fixed object, <u>as you</u> lift you chest "up".

It is **IMPORTANT** that you are drawing your shoulder behind you, <u>as you</u> lift your chest "up", (see left photo). If you don't draw the shoulder back, you will end up pushing it forward, (which collapses your chest muscles), which means you aren't getting a stretch, (see right photo).

Correct   **Incorrect**

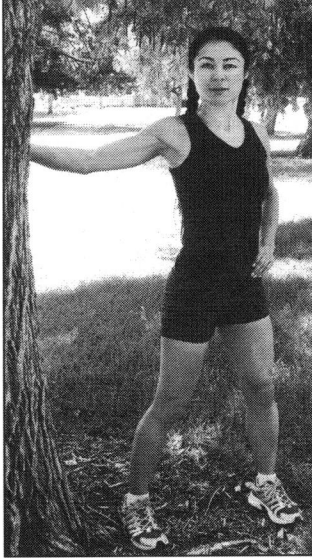
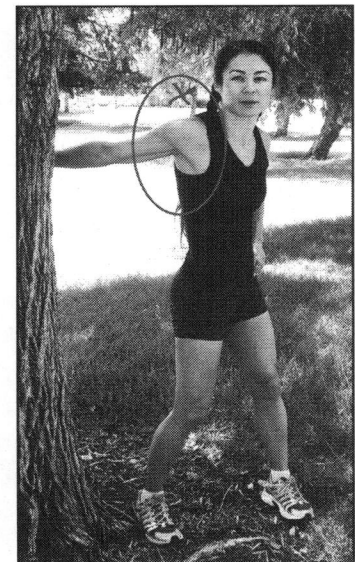

****

<u>Leg Ache</u>

Improve your posture

1. When you stand, make sure you do not lock your knees.
2. When doing exercises that require you to stand, make sure that your legs are hip/shoulder width apart.

Do **Elevate**:

If your feet/legs feel tired, and have a lot of pressure, then take the time at the end of the night to elevate you legs, (and during any time of the day when you get a few minutes here and there).

You can sit on the sofa and put your legs on a chair.

If you want to be a little more aggressive, then lay on the floor, and prop your feet up on your bed. *(Important Note: do not do this if you are past your first trimester of pregnancy)*

Stretches for your legs

Do **Leg swings**:

This helps increase circulation and flexibility in your legs.

1. Hold onto a doorframe, a tree, or fence. Have your body facing the fixed object.
2. Swing your leg across the front of your body, then swing it out away from your body. This should feel like a good stretch, not painful, so adjust your swing height accordingly. Also, keep your legs relaxed, so you can get nice active stretching.

Important Note: When pregnant, be very minimal with your "swing" across the front of your body.

Do this 10 times, then switch to the other leg.

(see photos on the next page)

Swing in   **Then swing out**

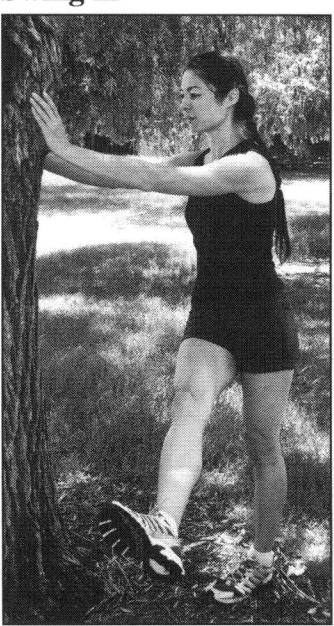 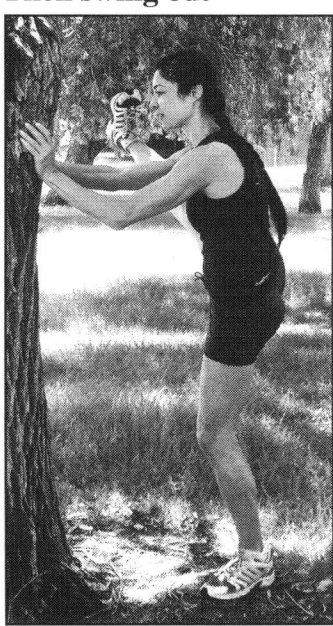

Do **Hamstring Stretch - Position 2 (hips pushed back)**

Note: This will be a similar stretch that you did earlier for your lower back.

1. You will use a chair, sofa end, bench, etc., as your stretching apparatus.
2. With your "standing leg", (the leg on the floor), make sure your foot is **parallel**, (turned out), to the object you are standing in front of. *(see left photo)*

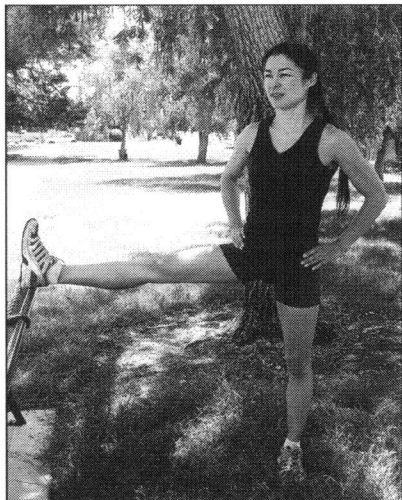 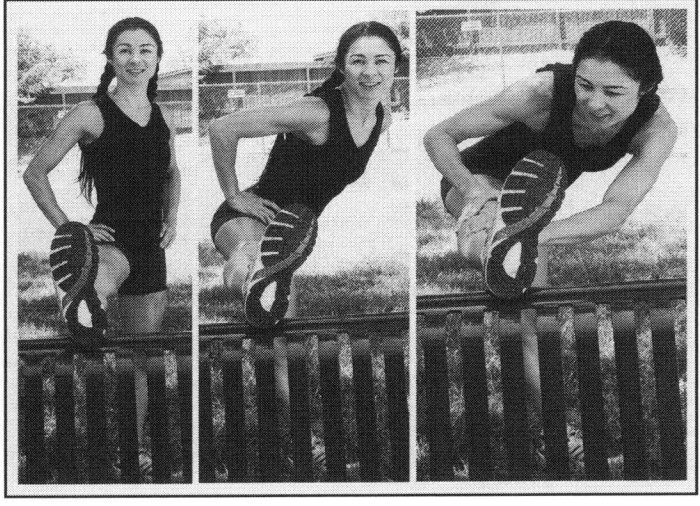

3. Lift a foot up onto the object you chose as your "stretching apparatus".

4. <u>Push you hips backwards</u>. This is an important detail to this stretch.

5. Lift your torso tall, and <u>gently direct your stomach towards your thigh</u>, and rest your arms onto your leg.

Important Note: Make sure that you only go as low as you can with your stomach LEADING the way.

Reminder: If you feel that you are off balance, make sure you have chair next to you so you can hold onto it if needed. If pregnant, you should always have a chair next to you for balance at all times.

Do **Leg Tendon Stretch** (foot forward, hip drops down):

Important Note: This will be similar to the other hamstring stretches, but please note the difference with the "standing leg" foot position; this detail is important.

1. You will use a chair, sofa end, bench, etc, as your stretching apparatus.

2. With your "standing leg", (the leg on the floor), make sure your foot is **FACING FORWARD**, (toes pointing to the object you are standing in front of. *(see photo below)*

Side View

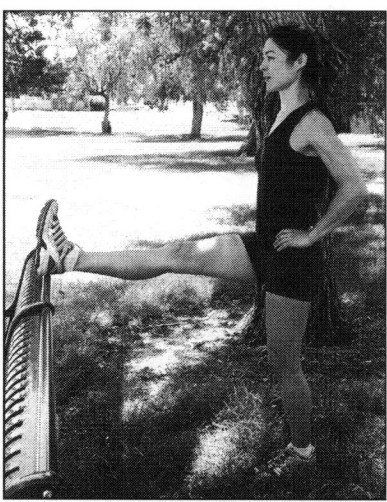

3. Lift the other foot up onto the object you chose as your "stretching apparatus".

4. Put both hands on your hips, then <u>turn your hips until they are level with each other</u>. This is an important detail to this stretch. *(see photos on next page)*

NOTE: *The hip on the side of the leg that is on the apparatus will be higher than the other side. <u>You want to turn the hip that is higher, down, by spinning it backwards and pushing it down.</u>*

Front View   (level by spinning the hip down)

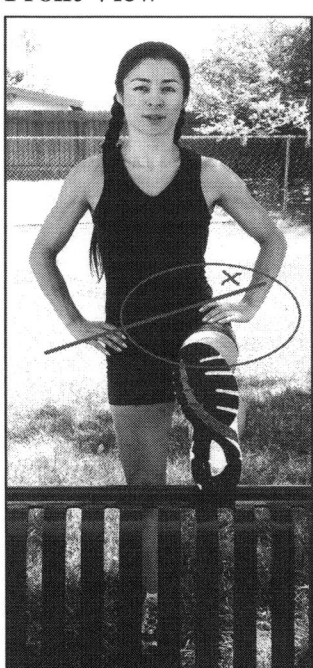 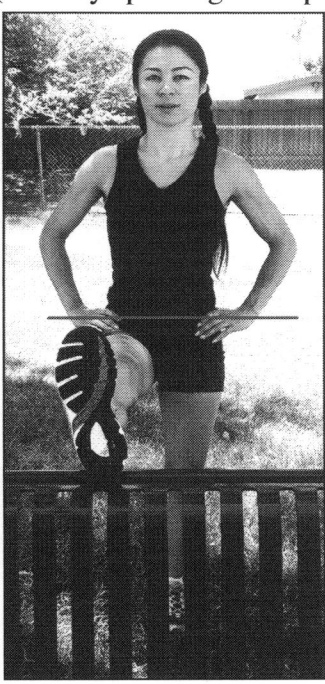

****

Feet Ache

Posture

Determine your foot strike…
Do you pronate? Do you supinate? What's the ideal posture then?

Well for everyone it looks slightly different, but if you are in chronic pain, then you probably can benefit from adjusting your feet strike. <u>Very often times, when you have feet posture that is not ideal, that contributes to causing feet pain, shin pain, knee pain, and even hip and/or lower-back pain. As well, very often times if you correct your feet strike, it can greatly reduce, or even eliminate those pains.</u>

My story: I pronate like most people, and it has caused me constant arch pain, calf tightness, and sharp knee pains for over 10 years of my athletic career. Especially with being an athlete, the constant repetitive motion of training was breaking me down faster than if I weren't an athlete.

With the help of orthotics, I propped up my feet for better posture, which in turn corrected the posture I had all through my legs, through to my lower back. While training with orthotics on, I was also strengthening my muscles, tendons, and ligaments in my feet/lower body, in this better posture. I eliminated all the pain I was experiencing in my arches and calves ever since, and it helped me manage my sharp knee pains. Now when I don't wear my orthotics, (when wearing flip flops or barefoot), I know where my foot positioning should be, in order to protect my joints and muscles. The orthotics saved my athletic career, and saved my joints and muscles.

<u>Despite having "normal" arch posture when looking at a foot, a person may still have issues for other reasons.</u>

Two common examples are:
1. There is a leg length discrepancy. This is very common, and the amount of problem that is caused depends on how much one leg is longer then the other, as well, how often and how intensely you are active.
2. Sometimes even if someone stands with "normal" arch posture, when that person starts moving, the arches change positions drastically.

Pronate:

This is very common. Pronating is when you apply weight on your feet, and your arches drop down; which then you can see your ankles and your knees turn inwards. Basically, pronating can affect your "posture" all the way up through your lower back, and even higher.

Stand in front of a mirror barefoot, and experiment with dropping your arches as much as you can, and lifting them up as high as your can. As you do this, watch how your ankles and knees turn in and out. You can also have a friend video you running, (front view), and then review the video.

Pronation in motion: Take a look at the photos below. The left photo is with the arches propped up properly and doing a squat, versus the right photo, with the arches dropping down and doing a squat. If a person does not have proper alignment when moving, (especially more rigorous movements), it causes a lot of joint, tendon, and ligament pain in the long run.

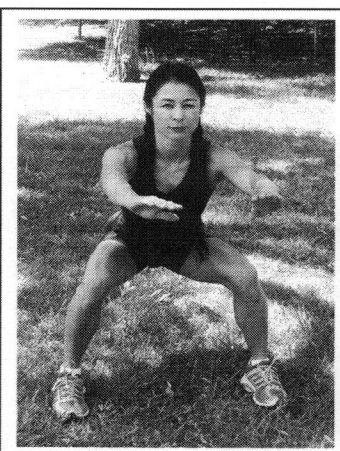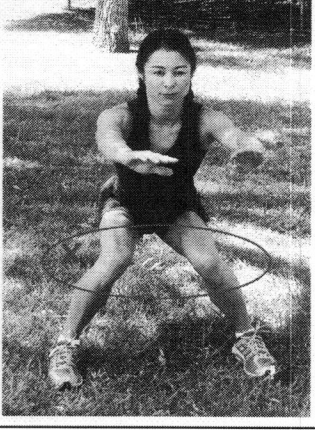

Supinate or high arches:

Supinating is when you put more weight on the outside edges of your foot. Supinating is not as common as pronating, but it can also cause problems because as with pronating, it alters the alignment of your body.

High arches are exactly as it sounds, higher than typical arches. Some people with high arches complain of pain as well.

A possible solution for pronating, supinating, and high arches is by wearing "hard" orthotics. Hard orthotics are plastic apparatuses that you wear in your shoes, and it helps support better alignment of your foot. Note: wearing common cushion inserts do not work well because they may not provide the necessary structural support, and also, they flatten too quickly.

There are several options for choosing where to get a pair of orthotics:

Custom:
A podiatrist, chiropractor, or similar specialist of orthotics, will take molds of your feet and create orthotics to exactly match the shape and size of each foot; they can correct any leg length discrepancy at this time. Correcting leg length discrepancies is a benefit of custom orthotics that you can't get with the over-the-counter pairs.

You need to go to a medical specialist for this type of orthotics.
Cost: Depends on your insurance and co-pay.

Over-the-counter (Dr Sholls):
If you go to DrScholls.com, click on their "Foot Mapping Center" icon to find a kiosk location near you.

The kiosk offers an you easy to follow, step-by-step process, that will measure your foot strike, and then it will tell you which type of orthotics from their selection is best for you.
Cost: around $50

Over-the-counter (Spenco):
Spenco makes many shoe insert products; make sure you get their hard plastic orthotics, rather than their many soft insert selections.

Popular locations: Sporting goods stores
Cost: about $29

Do **Elevate**:

This is the exact same recommendation as with leg aches.

Strength training for your feet

Do **Towel Scrunches**:

1. Sit on a chair that allows your feet to comfortably touch the ground.
2. Flatten out a hand towel on the floor, (long ways), in front of one of your feet.
3. Place your toes on the part of the towel closest to your body. Using your toes, start scrunching the towel until the part of the towel that's farthest from you, scrunches to you.
4. Do this 2 - 3 times with each foot.

Stretches for your feet

Do **Tennis Ball Massage**:

1. Sit on a chair that allows you your feet to comfortably touch the ground.
2. Place a ball under your foot, and roll your foot arch back and forth over the tennis ball. (Press down on the ball as hard as your tolerance allows).
3. Do this for a few minutes per foot.

Note: Too help add pressure on your massaging foot, use your hand and press down on the thigh/knee of the foot being massaged. You can also do this foot massage standing up.

Do **Toe Stretches**:

1. Stand bare feet with your feet shoulder width apart.
2. Keep one foot flat on the floor, and lift the other foot's heel up into the air WHILE pressing down on the ball of that foot, AS you continue lifting your heel up as high as you can.

You can do this exercise seated if standing creates too much pressure. Just make sure to <u>place the foot you want to stretch, slightly beneath the chair you are sitting in</u>.

Chapter Seven:

Skin Care

5 Things You Can Do For Preventative And Recovery Measures

1. <u>Use sunscreen</u>, use sunscreen, use sunscreen. Re-apply if exposed to sun for long periods of time, (this includes sitting by a window, which has you exposed to sun).

2. <u>Drink plenty of water regularly</u> - It is important to stay well hydrated. Your skin is considered the largest organ of your body, and it needs lots of water.

3. <u>Exercise</u> - Your blood circulation will be more efficient, carrying important nutrients throughout your entire body, including the skin. As well, the sweating is hydrating your skin from the inside out. Even 20 minutes on most days will make a positive difference.

4. <u>Use moisturizers in the evening</u> - Help keep moisture in your skin in two ways: One, the moisturizer will penetrate into your skin, and second, it will keep the outside negative elements from drying out your skin. Oils/moisturizer such as cocoa butter, aloe, jojoba oil, and sweet almond oil are hydrating, easily absorbed by your skin, and very affordable. *(Remember #1: use sunscreen during the day)*.

5. <u>Drink Green Tea</u> - Green tea is very good for the skin. It contains polyphenols, which according to recent studies, significantly increases circulation to skin. The mechanism isn't clearly known, but the thought is that if you are getting more blood flow to the skin, then the cells are getting increased nutrients, which can help support healthy skin.

Foods You Can Eat

<u>LEUCINE</u> rich foods - an amino acid that helps rebuild and tone skin: **Beans, Brown rice, Yellow corn, Lentils, Lean meats, Chickpeas, Nuts, Soy flour, Whole wheat**.

* <u>Our bodies do not create Leucine, it must be ingested</u>.
* Increases production of growth hormones.
* Recommended to patients after surgery to promote restoring of bones, skin, and muscle tissue.

LYCOPENE rich foods - which are high in antioxidants and helps build collagen: **Tomatoes, Watermelon, Grapefruit, Asparagus, Red cabbage**.

* Collagen boosts elasticity in skin.
* Antioxidants go after free radical. FYI: free radicals damage our cells and age us.

"**GOOD FATS**" – also known as Omega Fatty Acids, provide us with DHA and EPA: **Nuts and Fish**.

* Help metabolism.
* Have anti-inflammatory properties.

VITAMIN-A rich foods: **Sweet Potato, Carrots, Spinach**.

*Helps re-build tissues.

Supplements You Can Take

(Please consult with your doctor before adding supplements to your diet, especially if you are breastfeeding, or on medications).

Note:

1. Some supplements noted below are already included in your prenatal or multi-vitamin. Amounts in the prenatal or multi-vitamins are usually low, so supplementing additionally is usually safe, but for precaution, read labels, and talk to your doctor if you are pregnant or breast-feeding.
2. It is not a "make it or break it" if you don't get every single supplement listed here. If there are any concerns, (medical, financial, you simply don't want to take so many, etc), just pick the ones that you can take. The important thing is to stick with whatever you decide to supplement with for at least 3 months for the best benefits; constantly jumping from one thing to the next won't allow you to effectively see the results you are getting.

Essential or Important (with helping maintain and repair skin).

Primrose oil - contains linoleic acid, an essential fatty acid needed by the skin.
Coenzyme Q10 - improves cellular oxygenation.

Vitamin B - necessary for normal cell division and function.
Also known for anti-stress and anti-aging vitamins.
Vitamin E - promotes healing and tissue repair.
Selenium - encourages tissue elasticity.
Also know as a powerful free radical scavenger.

Herbs (helpful with maintaining and repairing skin).

Aloe Vera - topically used, has excellent soothing, healing, and
(pure) moisturizing properties.

Lavender - spray as a water mist on your skin throughout the day.
Make your own by adding a few drops of essential lavender oil in 4 ounces of distilled water.
Important Note: make sure you are using real lavender oil and not "fragrance" oil.

Breast Skin Care

It seems often enough, that when you hear a Mom mention something about their post breast-feeding breasts, it usually sounds unfavorable. This is an area, (along with stretch marks), where there is a "blind spot" of not being able to know the ultimate end result until after breast feeding.

There is still good news though…..

For most, your breasts will not be the same after pregnancy/breast-feeding, but remember, that DOESN'T necessarily mean it becomes "much worse". You can help lessen your breasts from having the stereotypical post-pregnancy/breastfeeding sagging, by applying simple preventative measures.

If you follow preventative measures, the end outcome is promising. Preventative measures are simple habit changes, and so there is no reason not to do them.

While Pregnant or Breastfeeding:

Wear a comfortable bra at all times, (day and night). You want to lessen the pulling of your breast tissues as much as possible, especially when there already is extra strain with added weight, and stretching at this time.

While exercising, always wear a regular bra underneath a jog bra for added support; even if you are just walking or doing light weight lifting, and even if you are an A or small B cup.

When breast feeding, make sure you support your baby "up" under you. While breast-feeding, you don't want your baby pulling down your breasts and unnecessarily stretching them. Your breast tissues are already being stretched from the increase in size for breast milk, the last thing you want to do is add to that pulling of tissue while breast feeding. You can easily prop "up" your baby with a blanket or pillow, so that way your arms aren't getting tired doing the lifting work. It's a simple adjustment that's easy to make, once you know this concept.

If using a breast pump, make sure you have the pump properly supported "up" under you. As mentioned above with breastfeeding, you don't want to have the breast pump pulling down your breasts. Again, it's a simple adjustment that's easy to make.

Try to limit breast engorgement by maintaining a very regular breast feeding/pumping schedule. When you first start breast-feeding, and when you wean your baby, you most likely will experience temporary breast engorgement, so limit the occurrences as much as possible in between those two phases.

After Breastfeeding:

Continue wearing a comfortable bra at all times, (day and night), for an additional year after you body has stopped producing milk.

After you stop producing milk and your breast size has "shrunk", your breast tissues are still contracting/tightening back for months after the initial obvious size has gone down. Keep your breasts supported "up", so it can shrink "up"; you don't want the weight of unsupported breasts limiting the "shrinking up" process.

It is also important to keep breast well supported during this time because the light compression also helps the skin contract.

Stretch Marks

As mentioned in the section "Breast Skin Care", there is a "blind spot" with stretch marks, with not being able to know the ultimate end result until after pregnancy/breastfeeding.

<u>What are they? What happened?</u>

Stretch marks are fine lines or streaks that appear on your skin that are caused by the fast changes that are occurring in the elastic supportive tissue, (dermis layer), that lies just underneath the upper most layer of your skin.

Since stretch marks represent a permanent change in the dermis (the deeper layer of skin beneath the surface layer), resurfacing cannot erase them. However, studies have shown that laser treatments can lessen the depth of stretch marks in some patients; the improvement rate has been shown to be between 20% and 50%.

Stretch marks most often appear on the stomach during the last trimester of pregnancy when the belly is growing the fastest, to accommodate the growing baby; some women also get them on their buttocks, thighs, hips, and breasts.

Stretch marks start out pink, reddish brown, purple, or even dark brown, depending on your skin color. They later fade, although they never totally disappear on there own.

Optional Treatments

<u>**Self-help:**</u> (home remedies/"Eastern")

Once stretch marks appear, unfortunately, there are not any natural solutions you can use to get rid of them completely.

Fortunately though, stretch marks do fade naturally over time.

In the mean time, you can use a **deep penetration oil based product,** and use this as you gently rub your stretch mark affected areas. This massaging can help with collagen and elastin stimulation, which in turn helps your skin rebuild itself faster.

<u>**Professional assistance:**</u> ("Western")

(There are always new technologies being created. Check with a professional for any new options, or modifications to the options listed below, instead of only relying on this book).

Important: Allow your body generous amount of months to heal on it's own before considering professional medical intervention. If your skin has not had enough time to heal on it's own, you can actually be hurting your skin more, by creating even more trauma and inflammation to it.

Note: Unfortunately with stretch marks, the torn dermal cells never fully recover, and although stretch marks are permanent, at least they can be made much lighter. Western remedies offer the fastest, most noticeable results when it comes to stretch marks.

Here are some of the options available:

Micro-Dermabrasion:

Uses tiny crystal beads to sandblast the skin, making the valley like areas of the skin to become worn out, and smoothing the skin out.

Some experts say the act of "peeling" does not work for stretch marks, others say it does. Where there is less controversy about micro-dermabrasion is that it is believed to jumpstart collagen production in the skin, which increases its elasticity, and helps it contract the marks into much thinner scars.

Laser: (examples: Fraxel)

Lasers are most effective on immature stretch marks that are still red in color.

Lasers work by penetrating the skin, and the light energy stimulates collagen, (which is a structural protein in our skin). Although you will not need as many treatments as with micro-dermabrasion, still multiple treatments will be required.

As noted on page 77, since stretch marks represent a permanent change in the dermis, resurfacing cannot erase them, however, studies have shown that laser treatments can lessen the depth of stretch marks in some patients.

Isolagen therapy:

A cosmetic procedure that uses your own cells to correct skin conditions. This procedure is a newer treatment approved by the FDA (Food and Drug Administration). The FDA recommends using Isolagen with other forms of treatment to improve stretch marks.

This process begins with a biopsy, typically taken from the back of your ear. The harvested cells are used in a laboratory to produce dermal fibroblasts, (fibroblasts are cells linked with maintenance, wound healing, and tissue metabolism). When sufficient quantity is created, portions of these cells are injected into the areas of your skin affected with stretch marks.

Typically it takes 3 sessions, with 2 weeks in between each session.

The reason that these fibroblast cells reduce the signs of skin abnormalities is still unknown. The FDA believes that these fibroblasts supply the dermis, (the layer just under the surface of your skin), with extracellular proteins that stimulate and strengthen the damaged collagen and elastin, reducing the appearance of the stretch marks.

Tummy Tuck (abdominoplasty):

This option is ONLY for stretch marks accompanied WITH moderate to severe loose skin.

Professionals note that since stretch marks cannot be "erased", that the only way to get rid of them is through excision, (cutting them out).

Tummy tuck surgery involves the removal of excess skin and fat from the middle and lower abdomen, and to tighten the muscle and fascia. *Fascia is a skin like sheet that the muscle attaches to.* There are two common types of Tummy Tucks, "Complete Abdominoplasty", and "Partial Abdominoplasty" (mini Tummy Tuck).

If a Tummy Tuck is the option you feel you may need to pursue, consult a licensed <u>board certified</u> plastic surgeon for all of the details and consultation on which type of Tummy Tuck would be best for your case.

Important: As with any surgery, it is recommended to get at least 2 to 3 opinions/recommendations.

Belly Skin Looseness

<u>What are they? What happened?</u>

Belly Skin Looseness is simply stretched out skin from when you were pregnant.

For many Moms, they have said to still see continued improvements with the tautness of their skin well after a year post-pregnancy. Some studies note that the skin continues to heal for up to 2 years after having a baby, to regain its full elasticity.

It is also normal to have skin look taut when standing up, but for it to sag, for example, when you are leaned over in a push-up position. Don't be so worried, especially within a year and a half of having had your baby; your skin is still "shrinking".

Just be sure that you are consistent with having well-balanced nutrition, because without proper nutrition supporting your skin's healing, how can you expect your body to heal properly. Also drink plenty of fluids, and get in some heart pumping exercise to circulate blood and moisture to the surface of your skin.

Optional Treatments

<u>**Self-help:**</u> (home remedies/"Eastern")

Wrap your belly

Wrap your belly every day and night for the first 1 – 2 weeks post-partum, (taking it off for a few hours here and there during the day, to allow your skin and wrap to breathe).

After the first couple of weeks, wear the wrap every night while you are doing the Ishio Method – Post Pregnancy Rehab Protocols TM, and most every night for the 1st year postpartum. It's highly encouraged for you to continue using the wrap occasionally beyond the 1st year postpartum.

Here are some of the belly wrap options:

Sillo Belly Wrap TM – Made specifically for use by post-pregnancy Mothers. <u>Brought to you by Michelle Ishio, and the Post Pregnancy Rehab Company</u>.

The **Sillo Belly Wrap** TM doesn't just "smash" your mid-section together, as with other popular belly wraps. The way you wrap the Sillo Belly Wrap TM around your body helps pull both sides of your 6-packs together.

Also, unlike other popular wraps, **Sillo Belly Wrap** TM is made of only soft cloth material without spines, so it molds very well to your body throughout the ENTIRE shrinking process. As you start shrinking and developing your waist again, it will NOT easily "spin" around your waist, or rise up to your ribs, like the other popular belly wraps.

*Important Note: For the first 13 weeks, you will wear the **Sillo Belly Wrap** TM crossing in the front of your belly, (to help close the "six-pack gap", while flattening your abdominal muscles). For the rest of the year, it's important that you wear the **Sillo Belly Wrap** TM crossing in the back, (to help smooth your skin, while continuing to flatten the abdominal muscles).*

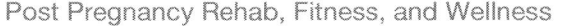

Listed below are other popular products that Mothers have used.

Belly Bandits ™ - Made specifically for use by post-pregnancy Mothers.

There seems to be as many Mothers loving these, as there are some Mothers taking note that they are stiff and sometimes hurts their ribs.

After the initial reduction in waist size due to normal shrinking post-pregnancy, many Mothers say that these do not fit the contour of their bodies anymore; that it rides up, spins around a lot, thus making them eventually unused-able for longer term use.

Belly Tauts ™ - Made specifically for use by post-pregnancy Mothers.
This is virtually a copy of the Belly Bandits ™. Similar reviews with them as well.

Over-the-counter medical abdominal braces - You can go to a pharmacy or on-line to get these.

What I'm talking about is not the exercise neoprene belly wraps meant for you to sweat, but the medical wrap meant for support; most often used after certain abdominal area surgeries.

These are not made specifically for post-pregnancy; they are made for various issues.

(Continued: Self-help for Belly Skin Looseness) Home Remedies/"Eastern"

Exercise regularly. At the very least, exercise the minimum suggested by the U.S. government, of 30 minutes total, for at least 3 days a week.

Heart pumping exercise of any kind will increase blood circulation, giving your entire body, (including skin), the benefits of oxygen and nutrients necessary for repairing. The sweat also helps moisturize your skin from the inside out.

Use deep penetrating oil frequently, for the first 6-weeks after having your baby, then use regularly throughout the first year post-partum. Oils such as jojoba oil is very healing for the skin, and absorbs well.

Baby Belly Jelly ™, (brought to you by Michelle Ishio, and the Post Pregnancy Rehab Company), is great during pregnancy, but also for post-pregnancy use as well. All of the ingredients in the **Baby Belly Jelly** ™ have anti-inflammatory and soothing properties, and are known for being quickly absorbed by the skin.

<u>Supplements</u> - Make sure you are at the very least, taking your pre-natal vitamins or multi-vitamins. The multi-vitamin can be like "insurance" to help make sure you are getting in a wide range of nutrients that are important for your body, (which includes repairing).

<u>Don't do excessive "dieting"</u> – You body needs nutrition to heal, and if you are cutting too many calories, (which then means important nutrients), your body will not have what it needs to properly heal.

Professional assistance: ("Western")

(There are always new technologies being created. Check with a professional for any new options or modifications to the options listed below, instead of only relying on this book).

Important: Allow your body generous amount of months to heal on it's own before considering professional medical intervention. If your skin has not had enough time to heal on it's own, you can actually be hurting your skin more by creating even more trauma and inflammation to it.

Laser Skin Tightening: (example: Thermage, Fraxel, Titan)

For mild case of loose belly skin.

Lasers work by penetrating the skin, and the light energy stimulates collagen, (which is a structural protein in our skin).

Laser skin tightening is said to give about 15 - 20% improvement in your skin's appearance. It's noted that some physicians say that lasers are unpredictable, sometimes giving great results, while other times the improvements are minimal.

The best thing to do is get an opinion for your personal body/belly by 2 or 3 professional laser technicians, and make a decision from there.

Tummy Tuck (i.e. abdominoplasty):

For loose belly skin that is moderate to severe. Most professionals agree that a tummy tuck gets the best results for moderate to severe stretch marks and loose belly skin.

Tummy tuck surgery involves the removal of excess skin and fat from the middle and lower abdomen, and to tighten the muscle and fascia. *Fascia is a skin like sheet that the muscle attaches to.* There are two common types of Tummy Tucks, "Complete Abdominoplasty", and "Partial Abdominoplasty" (mini Tummy Tuck).

If a Tummy Tuck is the option you feel you may need to pursue, consult a <u>licensed board certified</u> plastic surgeon for all of the details and consultation on which type of Tummy Tuck would be best for your case.

Important: As with any surgery, it is recommended to get at least 2 to 3 opinions/recommendations.

Pregnancy Mask (Malasma)

<u>What is it? What happened?</u>

Pregnancy Mask is a tan skin discoloration that is darker than your surrounding skin color. Although it can affect anyone, it is particularly common in pregnant women, those who are taking oral/patch contraceptives, or hormone replacement therapy medications.

The symptoms of pregnancy mask are dark, irregular color patches commonly found on the upper cheek, nose, upper lip, and forehead. These patches often develop gradually over time. Pregnancy Mask does not cause any other symptoms besides the cosmetic discoloration.

Pregnancy Mask is the temporary increase in your body's production of melanin, (the natural substance that gives color to hair, skin, and eyes). Excess melanin is triggered when exposed to sun.

Women with light brown to darker skin types are particularly more susceptible to developing Pregnancy Mask. Genetic predisposition is also a major factor in determining whether you will get this or not.

Usually the pregnancy mask fades within a few months after delivery and your skin returns to its normal shade, but for some woman, the changes never fully go away, and it becomes something they have to manage for the long term.

Optional Treatments

Self-help: (home remedies/"Eastern")

1. Wear broad-spectrum 30SPF sunscreen at all times during the day, and re-apply throughout the day.

2. Wear a hat whenever the sun it out and you are outdoors or driving. Even when you are in a building, you will want to create shade for your face if you are sitting near windows during the day

3. Eat tomatoes or grapefruits daily.

4. Make turmeric paste. Mix turmeric with lemon and water to create a paste, apply it to the affected areas of your skin, leave it on for 5 minutes, and then rinse. Turmeric helps inhibit the production off melanin in the skin.

5. Use a wash towel or soft exfoliating sponge, add a small amount of gentle face wash on it, and gently rub your face in circular motions, (especially the affected areas), to help get rid of the dead layers of affected skin. This speeds up skin turnover, but you still need to take preventative measures to keep the malasma from affecting your "new skin"; exfoliating alone will not get rid of the discoloration.

Professional assistance: ("Western")

1. Topical hydroquinone.

These ointment products usually have other ingredients in them to help peel the top layer of already discolored skin, for even faster results. **IMPORTANT: If you're pregnant or nursing your infant, don't use hydroquinone under any circumstances.**

Over-the-counter grade is typically 2%.

Some of the top rated over-the-counter products out there that you can buy:
pHaze 13 – Pigment Gel (2% hydroquinone)
Glytone Fading Lotion (2% hydroquinone)
Murad Rapid Age Spot and Pigment Lightening Serum (2% hydroquinone)

<u>Prescription grade</u> is at 4-8%.

Dermatologists recommend brands such as Lustra, Tri-Luma, and EpiQuin Micro, while other dermatologists manufacture their own line of hydroquinone.

There are conflicting reports on hydroquinone's safety; they say studies in rodents show some evidence that hydroquinone may act as a carcinogen, (cancer-causing chemical). Its cancer causing properties haven't been proven in humans, but it is always important to know all your risks before making any decisions.

2. Glycolic Chemical peels.

<u>Professional esthetician or dermatologist:</u>

There are different "depths" of chemical peels, so talk to your specialist on what strength would be best for your situation. Professional "peels" are usually 20-30% in strength.

<u>Over-the-counter:</u>

If you want a more gentle and gradual "peel" for your skin, then there are "at-home chemical peel" products available.

Over-the-counter peels shouldn't contain more than 10-15% glycolic acid. With consistent use over three months, it will diminish slight pigmentation as if you had a professional "light" peel.

According to some dermatologists/estheticians, the controversy with "at-home chemical peel" products is that the results are very minimal because typical drug store brands only have about 5% or less of glycolic acid. They also note that you have to be careful to not "burn" your skin.

If you purchase glycolic chemical peels on-line, you can get stronger strengths versus most of the glycolic chemical products you find in a drug store.

Some of the top rated over-the-counter products that you can buy <u>on-line</u>:
Glycolix Elite Facial Cream (15% glycolic acid) *they offer other strengths as well.
Glytone Over-night Cream (14% glycolic acid)
B Kamins Glycolic 10 (10% glycolic acid)

Important Note: what's being suggested is, you want to start with a lower dose glycolic acid content such as 10%, (so your skin can adapt and strengthen), then work your way up to the

15%. If you want to eventually use a stronger percentage of glycolic acid, (i.e. 20%), then go to a dermatologist for a prescription.

3. Laser skin treatments. (example: Fraxel)

Not only is laser technology good at erasing dark spots on your skin, it concurrently also improves the condition of your skin, including fine lines.

....

Important Note:

Everything just listed are great options for getting rid of your pregnancy mask discolorations, but remember, unless you wear a hat whenever you are out in the sun, and apply and re-apply sunscreen during the day, you will most likely re-develop the pregnancy mask.

After spending the time and money to get rid of the brown marks, you don't want to have to go through the same process over and over again because you didn't properly apply the preventative measures to keep them away.

Chapter Eight:

Stress Management - Relief

I. Manage/Eliminate Post-partum Depression

Please go to Chapter 9 – Post-partum Depression, *for details on post-partum depression, self-help, and resources on heading back towards a better direction.*

You can often enough hear me say, "I need a mood re-set". I'm referring to when you consciously do something to improve your over-all mood/energy on a particular day, for if you are having a rough day. This "mood re-set" concept also means to consciously do something to improve your over-all mood on a very consistent basis, for if you are in a rough patch in life, or for long-term depression management. If it means you need to "mood re-set" every day of the week, then do it, because you can't wait until the end of the week, or until you are having signs of a "mini meltdown".

As far as needing "mood re-sets", don't look at it as a weakness or something negative, because it is not; it is only positive that you are putting forth action towards self-awareness, betterment of yourself, and betterment of your life, so you should be proud of yourself.

Whatever positive actions you do that is working for your "mood re-set", I can guarantee will give you a sense of accomplishment, and raise your self-confidence. Be upfront with yourself, without judgments, and address any chronic symptoms you may be having that are making it hard for you to manage feeling consistently "all right", (which affects how you manage everything else in your life, and how you are relating to others).

Having depression will make managing stress extremely difficult, and it NEEDS to be addressed.

* This is real, and not "made-up" in your head.
* You can't just mentally "will it away", you have to do more.
* It is not your "fault".
* It does not make you a "bad" mother, or a "bad" person.
* It is much more common than most people think.

You shouldn't feel that you have no choice but to suffer through postpartum depression.

* If your baby blues doesn't alleviate after a few weeks, you may have postpartum
  depression.
* If you have suffered from depression/chronic low moods in the past before having
  a baby, you are at higher risk for postpartum depression.

II. <u>Manage Non-Reciprocated Energy And Eliminate Toxic Energy</u>

Awareness that you have the ability and responsibility to design the ambiance of your life is powerful wisdom to have; its creativity and productivity are endless.

Manage the wasting of your energy on people and situations that's not properly reciprocating back to you. It takes energy to create positive intentions for your life, maintain self-discipline, develop good habits, exercise, start "that" project, take care of each family member's unique needs, so do you really want to waste your precious energy on unnecessary people/situations that won't positively reciprocate back to your life? Choose wisely where you will apply your "fuel", and make sure it is being replenished in return.

This also applies with not having someone else's chronic negative energy filtering deep into your life. Science tells us that energy cannot be created nor destroyed, and it just transfers from one form to another. Energy comes in all forms, and for the sake of this section, we will focus on spiritual energy. Regardless of someone's exact belief system regarding spiritual energy, one basic thing that most can agree on is that when someone is in a great mood, (or a horrible mood), that people around them can "feel", (and sometimes absorb), the energy that that person is exuding. It is important to eliminate those people/situations that perpetually add their own toxic energy into our lives. For those you can't eliminate completely, it's important to understand that as individuals, we can manage how we choose to perceive, absorb, react, accept, filter, etc, the relationship we are a part of.

This concept of eliminating "toxic energy" also includes if the energy is coming from within us, in the form of anger or resentment at someone else or situation. As mentioned above, as individuals, we are the only ones who can effectively direct the "state" we are in by managing how we choose to perceive, absorb, react, accept, filter, etc, the circumstance we are a part of.

Yes, it is easier said then done, but the point is it can be done, and any change makes the next step in change easier than the last, and so forth. There are people, groups, teachings, and organizations, of many backgrounds, that offer direction, support systems, or ideas to consider. Knowing that you can customize your life's ambiance is an exciting, creative process, that can help manage or eliminate most stressors of you life.

Friends

Simply put, do you consistently feel rejuvenated after hanging out with or talking to your friend on the phone? If your friend isn't being a friend that contributes positive energy into your life, then the "friendship" needs to be either re-evaluated with both sides in full agreement with non-judgmental cooperation, or eliminated.

Now, are you being a good friend to a friend? If not, why? It also takes a lot of energy to not be a good friend; being jealous, spiteful, or dishonest, are all draining even if it's you doing it to someone else. If you are having difficulties such as just mentioned, with multiple friends, then it's probably something starting from within you; it will require your own honest and non-judgmental soul searching, realizations, and practice with becoming internally healthier. If it's one particular friend that's "triggering" something that's an uncommon occurrence in your life, then you will have to try and figure out why, then figure out from there if it's something you need to work on alone, address with your friend, or if the friendship even warrants being worked on.

Family

Same thing as with "friends"; do you consistently feel rejuvenated after hanging out with or talking to your family member? Again, it doesn't matter if they are negative about you, or just negative in general, because it's all very draining.

If certain family members are continually harsh, negative, judgmental, etc, towards you, then you need to acknowledge to yourself that nothing you do will make any difference to make it "stop"; constantly defending yourself is a waste of your energy. If you are not repetitively asking for help, or complaining about your life, and are at peace with your being and path, should it matter what their strong opinions are?

A simple "management" solution is to limit calling or seeing these particular family members. There are no universal "rules" that says how often you are "required" to see or talk to family members; every family is different, every situation is different, so don't complicate your life with the "man-made" conscious/subconscious expectations you may be having. Take yourself off "auto-pilot", and look at everything from a wider perspective; this will make it easier for you to be able to find a balanced answer/solution that fits your personal situation.

When you do see these particular family members, keep the conversation light, and leave it at that. Limit getting involved in "deep" conversations, and simply decide, does it really matter at the end of the day for that conversation/debate; doing this will help foster the ability to consistently grow the basic appreciation of "having and enjoying family", without having the "man-made" conscious/subconscious expectation of what level of "friendship" you are "supposed to have" with your family members. You are born into family without a "choice", (friends are "choices"), so naturally, we need to have more patience, flexibility, and creativity when relating to family.

It also helps if you take yourself off "auto-pilot" with your conscious/subconscious expectations of how relationships with each family member "should" be. It's important to realize that having strict preconceived beliefs will probably create conflict, which then probably means guilt or regrets of some sort later on. It helps to have confidence that family member relationships don't have to be one certain way or then it is not "okay" or it's "wrong", because continuing to try to force something that simply wasn't meant to be, will be miserable for the people involved, and it will not work.

After all that has been said and done, it helps if your don't get so overly concerned with the notion of "it's fair or not fair", or "so-and-so's family", and so on; it all really comes down to being, "it is what it is", and what are you going to do to remain peaceful, positively productive, and maintain stress management, despite whatever circumstances you may be a part of.

Once you have a healthier flow happening for yourself, it will be easier to see what "battles" are worth engaging in or not, and you will also more clearly understand that majority of the defending, explaining, or debating ultimately doesn't matter.

Children

Raising kids will always be stressful. We all want to raise our children to have a solid foundation to which they can root and grow their life; for them to be well balanced and successful with whatever it is they choose to pursue personally, and professionally.

What helps with managing stress with our children is for us to maintain our own emotional/mental management, (for F.Y.I, this can apply to any genre of relationship in our lives). It gets difficult to solve anything if we engage ourselves so deep into our child's emotional ups and downs, that we lose focus on the original purpose at hand, or are having a tantrum ourselves. We have to remember that our children are learning to have personal management by way of watching others, and we are the biggest influences with teaching them through modeling with our own personal management. Not only does our own emotional and mental management affect our short-term stress management with our children, but what we do now will determine how future differences with our adult children will be managed; you can call this "long term stress management".

Stranger's negativity

Often times getting too caught up eavesdropping, or judging, or giving your two-cents into an "argument" that you come across randomly in public is unnecessary, and draining. If you are at a place of stress, save your precious energy for productive and positive, thoughts and actions, for your life, and loved ones.

It also helps tremendously to be able to be more "easy going". There are so many examples I can pull from, but I will pick a common example.

Lets use "road rage" for an example: you are the one that accidently cut someone else off, and now that person is yelling profanities at you? Don't absorb it to the point that it's really hurting your feelings. If it was an honest mistake, (like I'm sure the angry driver has done to others plenty of times themselves), then know it's an issue they are having within themselves, and they just took it out on you. Be more "easy going", and it'll be easier to move on without it being absorbed into your system.

Lets say someone "cut you off"; it helps tremendously when you can just let it go. For those that this would consistently set-off a temper, seriously contemplate, why does it get you so upset? Is it a reaction from being on "auto-pilot", and you don't even have any specific thoughts on why you get that angry?

If you end up with thoughts or reactions that are unnecessarily "angry", then there probably is a need for honest and non-judgmental soul searching, realizations, and practice with becoming internally healthier; there are deeper explanations/motivations for the constant "angry" reactions.

The point in this section is, encourage your ability to be more "easy going" when necessary, because it helps with your stress management. It's not worth wasting the energy to get so angry over something so meaningless in the grand scope of your life's path, with more significant hardships, and triumphs.

(This space intentionally left blank)

III. **Thought Management**

Awareness that you have the ability and responsibility to design the ambiance of your life is powerful wisdom to have; its creativity and productivity are endless.

* Know that negative thinking is a subconscious and conscious bad habit, which means that it can be replaced with a good habit.

* Know that negative thinking has zero purpose.

Please go to **Chapter 9 – Post Partum Depression – "6 Things That Must Be Done Consistently - Thought Management"** for more detailed information.

IV. **Don't Be So Hard On Yourself**

Many Moms do this by way of comparisons with other Moms, comparison to their own Mom, or personal fixed ideals on what kind of Mom they were going to be, even before having children of their own.

When other Moms do things differently than you, it doesn't mean that theirs is a "right" or "wrong" way, or even that yours is the "right" or "wrong" way; it's just a "different" way. All that matters is that it is "right" for your family, (family schedule, family finances, family personality, your individual child). In relation to comparing yourself with your own Mom, times are different; different circumstance, different resources, and simply put, different person/family members.

Did you have fixed personal expectations with what kind of Mom you were going to be, and maintaining that level of ideal is over-whelming you? This is a good time to do some honest and non-judgmental personal assessments to calm your inner thoughts and feelings. You should contemplate on things such as: Where and how did you get your ideas on what a Mom "should be" like? For specific things you've been rigid on, what are those things symbolizing for you? If comparing so much with other Moms, why does it matter so much? What will happen if you didn't care so much? How will you function with fewer "caring burdens"?

Mom's Bit's and Piece's:

"My child's pre-school knew that I would most likely say "yes" to a volunteer request since I usually did. I was in over my head eventually, especially after the birth of my 2nd child. One day I

finally said "no", and it was such a relief and not as scary as I thought it would be. I am much happier, and my family gets a more patient Mom." Mary S.

"There is no way to be a perfect mother, and a million ways to be a good one." Jill Churchill

"A few bad days don't define me as a Mom. My kids won't fail 3rd grade because I wasn't able to read to them for 20 min on Sunday." Meagan S.

"My son is too old for naps, but I am too tired and cranky for him to not have one. We have something called "calm time"; basically its when he spends time in his bedroom playing by himself while he leaves me alone for a little bit. I used to feel guilty, but I realized that it builds independence for him, and sanity for me." Nancy H.

V. <u>Shake your Body, Shake your Brain, Relieve your Mind</u>

One of the BEST ways to manage the stress in your life is through physical activity...especially if having to manage depression.

Remember at the beginning of this section, I talked about "re-set"? <u>Exercise is one of the fastest ways you can get immediate relief from stress, and get that immediate "re-set"</u>. Unlike any medication, exercise also has <u>favorable "side effects"</u>: stronger body, sense of accomplishment, confidence booster, healthier organs, and a nicer physique.

Do you feel you are too busy to fit exercise into your day, and it is not priority? Then let me ask you this: how do you feel about your relationship with yourself, your life, and your body right now? Now, think about how they all inter-relate with each other. Then ask yourself honestly: why is it that you are not, or don't believe you should be, one of your priorities?

Think back to the last time you needed or wanted to buy something that you didn't have money for at the time, and you figured out a plan to gather the money, and find time to go buy it. What about the time you were the "under dog", and wasn't supposed to accomplish something, but you did anyway? These examples mean that it's already "in you" to get to a place of empowering yourself. My point is, when you really wanted or needed something before, you found a way to make it happen, and this is no different.

Don't let the word "exercise" overwhelm you either. Exercise for stress relief and general health does not have the strict criterias as if you are training for a specific sport, which means regular exercise is do-able for everyone. As far as stress relief, practically any form of moderate intensity movements for an extended period of time is considered "exercise"; from a heart pumping aerobics video, sets of jumping jacks/jump rope done at home, or even "crazy" full-out dancing in your living room with your kids. Lifting weights also can count, but make sure you aren't taking too much rest in between sets, and you aren't lifting too light of weights, because you need to have your heart pounding. Be very consistent, and "shake your body", "shake your brain", and you WILL "relieve your mind".

From the first day of starting an exercise program, you can immediately feel the "mood re-set", and sense of accomplishment benefits of exercising; so as a self-discipline booster for when you struggle to maintain self-discipline, re-call about how great you feel after an exercise session.

Exercise releases the feel good hormone endorphins. Physical activity helps increase the production of endorphins, (one of your brain's feel-good hormones). Although many people refer to it as the "runner's high", other activities other than running can produce the same affect. Exercise can also help "re-set" the other mood hormones, (dopamine, serotonin, etc).

Exercise is a confidence and esteem booster because it WILL give you a sense of accomplishment. Having that sense of accomplishment will release the hormone dopamine, (which gives people feelings of reward, happiness, and pleasure). You will also develop good habits that can cross over to accomplishing other things, which are additional confidence boosters.

Exercise improves sleep, which is often disrupted by stress, depression, and anxiety. With better sleep, your body and mind can handle stress better. Also, sleep is when our body repairs and re-sets itself.

Exercise helps you focus on something other than your "problems" for the moment. Focus on being in the moment of your exercise, whatever it may be. Focus on the movements that are required with your physical activity, (i.e. how your swimming strokes feel, concentrating on you kicking and punching form, playing tag with your kids and the laughing).

If you are training with a training partner, usually talk about non-stressful subjects, and if you must about a stressor, limit it to the positive takes on its remedies. Just make sure you keep consistently training rigorously, and not turn the training session into a coffee break.

After a fast-paced workout, (whether it be 25minutes or 45+ minutes), you'll realize that you had a mental break from all of your daily stresses. <u>With the help of the endorphins, (and other feel good hormones), your problem solving will come through with a fresher, more positive outlook.</u>

After exercising, you need to **stretch**. Don't forget to take deep breaths as you stretch.

110

You don't want to skip exercise days often, but at the very least, instead of out right skipping an exercise day, you should stretch; to enhance blood flow to the ends and surfaces of your body, help relieve stress, and take out any "kinks" in your body.

Stretching with deep breathing can be a form of meditation. It helps your heart rate slow down, and increases the oxygen supply to the brain. A breathing technique used in martial arts is to breathe in deep through your nose, and breathe out through your mouth; try breathing that way.

We don't just carry stress mentally and emotionally, we carry it physically too; by stretching, you are relieving a lot of physical stress, and by physically calming your body down, it will also help calm some of your emotional and mental stress.

Refer to Chapter 11 – Starter Fitness Program – Standard Stretching Routine.

Mom's Bit's and Piece's:
When I have a really lethargic day, I grab my kids, and we go for a much-needed walk/jog around a few blocks. I know it may mess up their cartoon watching or video game time, but I realize that they can always go back to whatever they were doing, and exercise is important for them too. A little sacrifice for a Mom who always sacrifices for them is perfectly fair.
Shelly A.

VI. Your ZZZZZZ's Do Important Things

Sleep is when our body recovers from everything it went through during the day, (mental, emotional, and physical).

During REM sleep, our body produces the hormone serotonin. Serotonin is the hormone that helps create a sense of well-being; it is one of the main hormones that regulate our mood. The body does not store serotonin, and it must be created daily.

Without proper sleep, our immune system also lowers; our body doesn't heal as effectively, our memory is impaired, we are more accident prone, etc, and all of these create stressful situation.

If you are not getting enough sleep, it is important to figure out a way to increase sleep and/or get better quality sleep, (even with the challenges of a new baby, because it's that important). Be creative. Be disciplined. It's important that sleep gets figured it out.

(Read some suggestions on the next page).

Optional Treatments

Self-help: (home remedies/"Eastern")**...for sleep**

1. Keep as consistent of a sleep schedule as possible: Go to bed within the same hour each night, and wake up within the same hour as well.

2. Establish a bedtime ritual: Just like you would read to your child before bedtime to signal that it is soon time for bed, create a ritual for yourself.

A great ritual is a nice 5 minutes slow stretching routine while breathing deeply. Not only is it good for your body, it is good for your brain. As mentioned before, we don't just carry stress mentally and emotionally, we carry stress physically too. By stretching, you are relieving a lot of your physical stress, and by physically calming your body down, it will also help calm some of the mental and emotional stress.

3. Lavender Aromatherapy: Studies have proven that lavender aids in sleep. Put droplets or spray the inside of your pillowcase for maximum effect.

Important Note: Be sure to get REAL lavender oil or spray, (aroma therapy grade). It is the properties in essential oil that makes the difference, not simply the manufactured smell of synthetic lavender.

4. Increase Tryptophan in your food regimen: Tryptophan is an amino acid found naturally in the foods that we eat. Tryptophan increases serotonin in the brain. Serotonin is the natural compound that promotes feelings of well-being and relaxation. A serotonin deficiency can result in sleep disturbances, anxiety, depression, and a propensity to overeat.

Food Rich in Tryptophan: (healthiest foods easily available, and listed from highest to least) Chicken, Soybeans, Turkey, Tuna, Lamb, Salmon, Halibut, Shrimp, Cod, and Sardines.

5. Calcium and Magnesium Supplements: Take calcium supplements about 1 hour before going to bed.

Calcium is known to be a sleep booster, and when taken with Magnesium, it is known to be more effective. Most calcium supplements come with the option of having the magnesium included.

We need to make sure we get in our calcium everyday anyway, so we can get two things taken care of at once.

Note: As of right now, the recommended calcium intake for females between the ages of 11 - 24 years of age is 1500mg a day, women aged 25 - 50 years of age is 1000mg a day, and pregnant and nursing women is 1200 - 1500mg a day.

IMPORTANT NOTE for the next few self-help options for sleep:

<u>Do Not Use Them While Pregnant or Breastfeeding</u> – contradictions are not well known. Always consult with your doctor before adding any supplement/medication. Everybody has a unique body, and taking different supplements/medications, which means everyone's needs or risks are different.

When it comes to the supplements listed on the next page, **only try one remedy at a time** so you know which remedy is working for you, as well, you are not "over dosing" your body. Try each remedy for at least 2 - 3 months before deciding whether it is working effectively enough or not, and switching to another remedy.

(Continued Self-help for Sleep) Home Remedies/"Eastern"

6. Guna Sleep *(registered trademark)***:** Featured on the Dr. Oz TV show. Dr Oz invited a pain management specialist on his show to talk about his patients who have trouble sleeping because they are experiencing pain.

The pain management specialist works with a lot of athletes and moms who are experiencing pain and insomnia, and he said that Guna Sleep helps his patients get a restorative nights sleep. Dr. Oz also said that Guna Sleep has been so effective that many of his patients have been able to get off of their sleep medications, which often has undesirable side effects.

You take 20 drops under the tongue, 20 minutes before going to bed.

7. Wild Lettuce Supplement: Not only is this known to calm restlessness and reduce anxiety, wild lettuce supplement can be good for headaches, and muscle or joint pain.

The typical dosage of wild lettuce supplement is 30 - 120mg before bed. Keep the dosages as low as possible.

8. Hops Flower tea: This is a flower used in beer making. It is known for its calming effects. This extract has been widely used as a mild sedative for anxiety and sleep problems.

Typical dosage of Hops would be 30 - 120mg before bed. Keep dosages as low as possible.

9. Valerian Capsules or tea: Valerian is a popular herb used throughout Europe. This herb is known to increase the amount of time you spend in deep sleep and REM sleep, (rapid eye movement). This herb is used to soothe anxiety and relax active minds. Valerian is most effective when used over a long period of time. Only drawback for some is the odor with teas.

Typical dosage for Valerian is 200 - 800 mg before bed..

Precautions: For a few people, Valerian can be more stimulating then calming; usually lowering the dosage eliminates this problem. Also avoid Valerian when you are pregnant.

10. Melatonin supplement: Melatonin is a hormone, (that your body naturally produces), that tells your body when it is time to sleep. This is an over-the-counter supplement, but it is a hormone, so ask your doctor before taking this supplement.

Research is showing that melatonin supplements have improved sleep in individuals, however, taking too much can give you side-effects such as waking up with a "hung-over" feeling, and eventually with long-term/too high dosage use, your sleep cycle will be impaired.

Melatonin usually comes in 3mg doses, and since your body naturally only produces around .03 - 1.0 mg of melatonin, you want to take the least amount possible; so what you want to do is bite a small fraction of the pill, and discard the rest. *Important Note:* Melatonin is not for long-term use.

Professional assistance: ("Western")...**for sleep**

(There are always new options being created, so check with a professional for any new options, instead of only relying on this book).

Note: Over-the-counter or prescription sleep aids may help when temporary stress, travel, or other temporary disruptions keep you awake. If you have chronic sleep issues, the best approach is to use "lifestyle change" and/or "natural" remedies.

Important Note: Talk to your doctor before taking any over-the-counter sleep aid if you are currently, or very recently have taken any drugs for depression or other psychiatric condition, as well, drugs for any other specific condition. It is not recommended to take any of these sleep aides when pregnant or breast-feeding.

1. Over-the-Counter Sleep Aides: Most of these medications contain antihistamine, which cause drowsiness.

Here are some common over-the-counter name brand sleep aides:
Sominex
Benadryl
Tylenol PM

2. Over-the-Counter 5-HTP Supplements: Many experts believe that tryptophan deficiency may cause you to have problems with your sleep. 5-HTP is made from tryptophan, and it helps the body make serotonin. Having low serotonin levels are known factors for causing sleeping problems. Low levels of tryptophan are most common with people who are depressed. If your sleep problems are associated with depression, then it would be important to ask your doctor about 5-HTP, to find out if you have low levels of serotonin or contradictions with taking 5-HTP.

Important Note: There is conflict with 5-HTP if you are currently using an anti-depressant; taking both 5-HTP and an anti-depressant may cause you to have too much serotonin, (serotonin toxicity). Because 5-HTP has not been thoroughly studied in higher end clinical settings, possible side effects and interactions with other drugs are not well known.

Refer back to the "Self-help for sleep" section above; to first try foods as a way of increasing tryptophan, rather than going straight to taking 5-HTP.

3. Prescription Sleep Aides: (Non-Benzodiazepine / Benzodiazepine / Rozerem)

Non-Benzodiazepine

In recent years, a newer class of sleep medications has been developed. These medications are often referred to as "non-benzodiazepine", or "benzodiazepine receptor agonists". These newer medications seem to have better safety profiles, less adverse effects, and are also associated with lower risk of dependence, abuse, and negative withdrawal, in comparison to the "benzodiazepines". Other advantages of non- benzodiazepines medication are not having the "hang-over" effect the next day.

Non-Benzodiazepine medications:
Ambien (Zolpidem)
Sonata (Zaleplon)
Lunesta (Eszopiclone)

Although these medications are safer than the benzodiazepines, it is not recommended that they be used on a long-term basis either, (with the exception of Lunesta). Lunesta has been approved by the FDA for longer-term use.

Benzodiazepine

The "benzodiazepines" have been the most commonly used medications for the treatment of insomnia, and are definitely safer than older sleeping medications, (i.e. barbiturates: Amytal, Nembutoal, Seconal).

Benzodiazepines are only recommended to be used on a short-term basis since physical tolerance and dependence can develop. In addition, these medications can often produce a "hangover" effect the following day. These medications are being mentioned in this book since they are options that are available, although I don't recommend these as a "go-to" option.

Benzodiazepines medications:
Klonopin (Clonazepam)
Ativan (Lorazepam)
Xanax (Alprazolam)

Rozerem (ramelteon)

Razerem works by mimicking melatonin, (a naturally occurring hormone that is produced during the sleep period).

Rozerem may have advantages over the benzodiazepine and non-benzodiazepine classes of medications because it specifically targets the brain structure that is responsible for the sleep-wake cycle. It is the first medication that does not show evidence of dependence, abuse, and is approved by the FDA for long-term use in adults.

Important Note: *For more detailed information of each medication and it's side effects, and/or recommendations specific for you, please consult your primary care physician.*

VII. <u>Don't Lose Yourself</u>

Losing yourself creates at the very least, a subconscious level of stress.

We were someone before we were Moms; becoming a Mom should just ADD to who we are, and NOT replace it.

If we lose our individuality and make our "be all and end all" become our children, (even our partner), then when it's not going smoothly with these people for whatever reason, then our happiness will be in complete control of other people, and not ourselves.

Awareness that you have the ability and responsibility to design the ambiance of your life is powerful wisdom to have; its creativity and productivity are endless.

It is extremely important that we know how to feel fulfilled as individuals standing alone, if we are to take responsibility for our life without excuses. Whether you were properly fulfilling yourself as an individual pre-children, or you need to re-invent yourself because you didn't have it quite right even at that point, the objective is that the concept is something that's important to strive for.

It's not to say that our family can't be a big part of us feeling fulfilled and happy, but it is just as important that we can do that for ourselves without anyone else involved. **We need to have a "go to" place that's uniquely ours, to recoup, resolve, and recapture effectively.**

"When I have time to do things I enjoy, I'm calmer.
Dealing with tantrums is rough when you want to join them".
Amber

If you had a serious hobby such as painting, running 5K's, or anything in between, then schedule that into your family structure. Grant it, you won't be able to spend as many hours participating with it as you did before, but you can figure out a way to maximize the time you can dedicate to it at this point in your life. If you don't have anything in mind that you want to get back to, then find something you were always curious about, something that is positive, just for you, for your individuality. The point is, if it is something you always found important and was part of your identity before you had children, then don't let it disappear...don't let yourself disappear.

The children will be supportive.

You will be a good role model by having the children grow up in an environment where it's "normal" to go beyond the minimum requirements of life.

It should be "normal" to sacrifice for Mom, as it is for Mom to sacrifice for the children.

Have an adventurous time continuing you, or reinventing yourself!

"Be not afraid of growing slowly, be afraid only of standing still."
Famous Chinese proverb

VIII. <u>Say "No" To Strict Dieting</u>

Nutrition affects your hormones, your hormones affect your energy and mood, your energy and mood affects how you view life, and how you view life affects how live life.

Please take having consistent, healthy nutritional lifestyle habits into high consideration, if you don't already do.

When I say "nutritional lifestyle habits", it doesn't mean you have to eat "perfectly" all the time; it's a lifestyle habit with at least 80% healthy, and 20% flexibility. Go to <u>Chapter 5 – Nutritional Guidance</u>, so you can understand the basic guidelines, and personalize a simple plan that's easy enough for you to start and maintain.

Here are some basic concepts of well-balanced nutritional lifestyle habits:
* An array of food groups with each meal, (with leafy and colorful vegetables dominating the plate, and meats at about your palm size).
* Portion control, (which includes not over-eating AND as importantly, not under-eating).
* Figure out how many "junk food/dessert" calories you have available to consume a day, and stick with that number on most days.
* Drink mostly water, (over juices and sugar drinks), because they count as part of your "junk food" calorie alottment a day. Would you rather drink or eat your "junk food" calories?

Disclaimer: If you have specific health concerns or needs, then what your doctor/specialist tells you will supersede what's written in this book.

IX. <u>Tilt Your Lips Up, Tilt Your Eye Brows Up</u>

When you are constantly slightly frowning, and your eyebrows are sitting low and looking stressed, you are reinforcing the hormones associated with that mood. By chronically having that type of facial expression, it's basically your "default" face, the face you make when you are relaxed and not paying attention; it's the person that the "world" sees and responds to consequently.

Our bodies will hormonally react to what our physical bodies are going through, so can that include physical facial expressions? <u>Can a subconscious and constant "default facial expression" trigger a constant flow of hormones specific to the mood that that facial expression represents?</u>

Looking at it from this angle: there was a study done, where through science, they are proving that our thoughts affect us on a cellular level. If that is the case, and there is a "bridge" like that open, then why can't "traffic" flow both ways? So then in reverse, on a more grand cellular level, by physically smiling, frowning, etc, can we affect our thoughts, which can affect our hormones?

Regardless of any scientific data, or my theory, try this.....

Slightly smile AND raise your eyebrows up a tad; do you feel instantly "lighter"?

When you are in a good mood, make a conscious effort to frown for a few minutes. Do you feel any change in mood, or mood-like sensation?

When you are tired and have some time left at work, or your kids are challenging your patience all day, "turn your lips up" and maintain a very slight smile to offset some of the mood you are experiencing; remember to slightly raise your eyebrows too. It might seem awkward at first, especially if you are upset, but it will relieve some of that tension. Doing this is so subtle that no one can see that you are doing this, so give yourself a breather, and get rid of some tension.

After all that has been said, (and concepts that may be challenged), at least what many can agree on is that whatever we are showing on your face can affect how people interact with us, with the potential to make our day better or even more difficult. With this concept alone, it makes it worthwhile to take into consideration, and adjust our "default facial expressions" if needed.

X. <u>Watch stand-up comedians</u>

Laughing does make a major difference with stress management; it triggers "feel good" hormones. Laughing also activates the muscles associated with happiness, (i.e. smiling), which also helps trigger the feel good hormones.

Go see a live stand-up comedy show. This helps you break your routine, gives you a break from your kids, and you will also be surrounded by other people in laughter, out to have a good time.

If going out is not possible for whatever reason, rent a DVD, or go online and stream a movie to your computer; any comedy will do.

Even if you "don't feel up to it", watch comedy anyway, and you won't be able to help but smile. When you see that it works, you will watch again without the hesitation you may have had the first time. I say comedians are like our health care professionals too!

XI. <u>Play with Bubbles</u>

Bubbles are meditative.

Keep a little bottle in you car; you never know when you can take that 5 min break to play.

While you watch the bubbles floating away every which way so peacefully, <u>breathe deeply</u> to slow down your pace. If you have access to music from your cell phone, or your car, <u>play some relaxing music</u> while you meditatively play.

This is a relaxing bubble ballet show just for you.

XII. <u>"Rescue Spray"</u> *(registered trademark)*

Homeopathic remedy derived from various flowers.

This product was featured on Dr. Oz TV show. It is derived from a group of flowers that have been known to ease stress and anxiety.

It is safe for children and adults. It comes in sprays, pastilles, and gum.

It was noted that before the inventor of this product passed away, he begged that the formula not be changed; it is still the original formula and has not been changed since its invention over 70 years ago.

Many medical professionals insist that this works for their patients.

Chapter Nine:

Postpartum Depression

Baby Blues?

After having a baby, Moms have hormone shifts that sometimes cause her to have low moods; one part of the day she feels happy, and another part of the day she feels like crying. You may feel a little depressed, having a hard time concentrating, losing your appetite, or find that you can't sleep well even when your baby is asleep.

It's noted that as much as 80% of Moms get a bout of baby blues. Symptoms usually start a few days after delivery, and may last several days or a couple weeks; baby blues are considered a normal part of early motherhood.

Could It Be Postpartum Depression?

Postpartum depression (PPD) feels more severe then baby blues, as well, it tends to last much longer.

PPD can appear within days or even months after childbirth, and often times lasts for months, and even longer than a year if not properly treated as needed. It is estimated that about 10% of Mothers may develop post-partum depression.

Post-partum depression is more likely to appear if you had any of the following:

* Previous depression not related to pregnancy
* Severe premenstrual syndrome (PMS)
* Difficult and very stressful marriage/relationship
* Difficult pregnancy or delivery
* Stressful life events during or after childbirth, (such as death in the family, abrupt financial difficulty such as a job lay-off, major move, etc.)

Post partum depression is treated much like any other depression, with counseling and/or medicines. Exercise is critical and highly encouraged, and it is important to have a support system of family/friends.

Symptoms Of Postpartum Depression Through Mom's Words

(you do not have to experience all of these symptoms to have PPD)

* Feeling chronically overwhelmed. You feel like you can't handle being a mother. May be wondering whether you should have become a mother in the first place.

* Feel irritated or angry often. Patience is limited. Feel resentment towards your baby or your partner. Anger may feel out-of-control.

* Feel guilty. Believe you should be handling motherhood better. Feel like your baby deserves better. Wonder whether your baby would be better off without you.

* Having trouble or are not bonding with your baby.

* Feel empty. You are just going through the motions.

* Regardless of how much you try, you just can't understand why you are feeling the way you do.

* Feel deep sadness. May cry often.

* Feel hopeless. You wonder if you situation will ever get better.

* Aren't hungry, or the opposite, and the only thing that makes you feel better is to eat.

* Sleep is all mixed up. You can't sleep when your baby sleeps. Have trouble falling asleep at night, or if you manage to fall asleep, you often wake up in the middle of the night, then can't go back to sleep. Maybe all you want to do is sleep even if it's neglecting some necessities. Maybe you don't want to go to sleep. You simply know that your sleeping is very messed up, and you know it's not just because of the new baby's schedule.

* It's hard for to concentrate. It's hard to focus. It's hard to remember what you were supposed to do. It's hard to make a decision.

* Feel disconnected from everyone for some reason. There is you on one side of the wall, and everyone else on the other side.

* Refer to your self as the "you from before" and "you, now".

* Feel something is "off", so you make sure you are doing many things "right" for yourself. You are exercising. You are eating healthy and taking vitamins. You are engaging in conversations with your friends. You are constantly referring to positive thoughts to help counter your negative feelings, but you just don't seem to be consistently "getting over it".

Having depression makes everything "harder", and it NEEDS to be addressed.

* This is real, and not "made-up" in your head.
* You can't just mentally "will it away", you have to do more.
* It is not your "fault".
* It does not make you a "bad" mother, or a "bad" person.
* It is much more common than most people think.

You shouldn't feel that you have no choice but to suffer through postpartum depression.

Getting To A Better Place

For those struggling with depression/chronic low-moods, you have to focus on consistent over-all health management rather than one particular thing, if you want to have real and long-term successful mood management; this means your sleep, balanced nutrition, stress management, socialization, thought management, and physical activity.

When struggling with depression, managing over-all health may sound and/or be over-whelming, however if you take it step by step, (regardless of how small or large each step is), the point is that you will always be in a better place guaranteed, than if you just "give up", and choose to allow life to stagnate where it is.

The being "caught in a rut" state is very stubborn, so it's important for you to constantly remind yourself that, one, it is a choice to try "nothing" while sitting in this rut, two, bad habits that hold you back can be modified, and three, the hard work with putting into practice of modifying your lifestyle/bad habits does work, and will "gift" you for a lifetime.

Good news is that doing something "simple" from each "category" is a sufficient start; don't take too big an initial leap because it will create an overwhelming transition. It's important to write down, with simple bullet points, your plan for yourself, and hang it up somewhere that you can see it daily. Writing the simple bullet points will help you "solidify" it better in your conscious and subconscious, and make it more real for you. It's also good to know that everything doesn't have to be done "perfectly", and as long as you are doing 80% of everything you set for yourself, on an 80% consistent basis, you will feel abundantly better with healthier habits that can remain with you for a life-time.

Discipline is commonly the hardest factor when developing/modifying habits, so with that said, once you decide what habits you need to have as a part of your daily life, your **primary focus** needs to be to **very frequently verify your purposes/intentions** for this journey your are taking.

"Authentic commitment to your purposes and goals...
Discipline, appropriate Character traits, and Perseverance will follow.
The Courage to "dare to be" shines brighter than you even imagined possible."

It helps some, to take the "emotion" out of the process for a bit, and to simply "do" what's on the "short list of expectations" that is set for the self. If this isn't the "trick" for you, that's OK, but point is, you need to acquire a "go-to" that works for you, (and do it ASAP), because guaranteed, you will need to fall back on it many times.

Moms With Postpartum Depression Found These Things Helpful

*Find someone non-judgmental to talk to, and tell that person about your true feelings.

*If at all possible, get in touch with people who can help you with childcare. This support will help you find time for yourself so you can get your needed rest, and find time to do something special to take care of yourself.

*Know that you aren't "weak" because you feel overwhelmed. Being overwhelmed is normal; don't be hard on yourself because you feel that way.

*Don't try to be a "supermom" all the time. Be honest about how much you can do, and ask other people to help you when you need it. It's OK to tell people "no" when they ask for favors too. Also remember that things don't have to be done "perfectly.

*Find time to do something for yourself, even if it's only 15 minutes a day; try reading or taking a bath.

*Write down your thoughts and feelings. This is a way for you to vent without any judgment. Once you begin to feel better, you can go back and re-read your diary, and it will show you how much better you have gotten, and remind you for the next time you are in a rough spot, that things always can get better.

*Find a support group in your area. Support makes a world of a difference.

*Don't hesitate to talk with your doctor about how you feel; that is what they are there for.

---

6 Things That Must Be Done Consistently For Depression Management

<u>Self-help:</u> (home remedies/"Eastern")

1. You Must Exercise

There is no compromising this; exercise works for immediate relief, and long-term management.

Exercise is vital for mood stabilizing. Unlike any medication, exercise has <u>favorable "side effects"</u>: stronger body, sense of accomplishment, confidence booster, healthier organs, and a nicer physique; no pill can give you that.

Many have heard about the "feel good" hormone, "endorphins", that is released when exercising, but the depression management that exercise offers is more than that. Although not quite clear, exercise is most likely helping all of the mood neurotransmitters to function better in general, thus helping with over-all mood management for the longer-term.

It is critical that you help regulate your mood hormones. When you are in depression or low moods, it is hard to get going, but you must do something rigorous for 20 minutes or more. When you see that it DOES WORK, you will have less resistance the next time it's time to exercise. Recalling how much better you felt all the other times you found a way to get yourself going with exercise will make maintaining discipline much easier, and help create your good habit.

Don't let the word "exercise" overwhelm you either. Exercise for stress relief and general health does not have the strict criterias as if you are training for a specific sport, so regular exercise is do-able for everyone.

After an easy warm-up, make your exercise more rigorously. Start exerting yourself, alternating between 50% and 80% effort, so the feel good hormones will be triggered more quickly; this training intention is especially useful for when short on time. Afterwards, make sure you wind down your mind and body, and stretch for a few minutes when you are done.

Exercise is a big part of depression, stress, and sleep management. Please go to Chapter 11 – Starter Fitness Programs, for exercise programs you can do anywhere, at no cost. Go to Chapter 8 – Stress Management/Relief - Shake your Body, Shake your Brain, Relieve your Mind, for a little more insight about exercise and stress relief.

2. Thought Management

Awareness that you have the ability and responsibility to design the ambiance of your life is powerful wisdom to have; its creativity and productivity are endless.

1. Know that negative thinking is a conscious and subconscious bad habit, which means that it can be replaced with good habits.

2. Know that negative thinking has zero purpose.

Reduce the amount of negativity in your life. As I mentioned in Chapter 7 – Stress Management/Relief, eliminate toxic friends, and keep communication with toxic family members to the bare necessities; it doesn't matter if they are negative about you, or just chronically negative in general, because it's all very draining. Also don't watch the news so much, or TV shows and movies with stressful story lines, (for the time being anyway), because often times when a person is struggling with negative thoughts/feelings, news and entertainment shows often times end up becoming a "confirmation" of the negative thought processes.

Negative thoughts need to be shifted away immediately. When it first starts coming on, you have three ways you can immediately handle it.

First way is more basic, and it is good for when you are first learning to let-go of negative thoughts. What you want to do is divert your though process to anything simple, yet pleasant around you. You want to get in the habit of not allowing yourself to have negative thoughts constantly running through your head.

Second way requires more thinking, but it's a better technique than the first. Immediately replace the negative thought with a positive one; even if the thought seems far-fetched at the moment, just do it, because you are trying to break the bad habit of negative thoughts sabotaging you.

The third way requires the most energy, but gives you the confidence of understanding yourself more, and having more skillfulness with your life. This is good for once you are able to face your negative thoughts without judgment, and you have full conviction that the way you've been processing thoughts doesn't benefit you at all. What you do is acknowledge what your negative thoughts are, then without judgment, and in simple form, consider why it pops into your head the way it does. The next step, (which takes multiple efforts), is to identify your belief/thought system that encourages those negative thoughts, so as to initiate a positive transformation from the root of where it's coming from. You will need to challenge your current subconscious belief/thought system if you want to successfully be able to "program" a new belief/thought process. *FYI: some can do this on their own, while many others need a support system; which one you choose should be the one that gets the best action oriented progress out of you.*

Reflect on things you like about yourself, like about your life, and look forward to in the future. There are good things, so don't take the "lackluster route" by simply saying, "There is nothing". This list doesn't need to be long, even if only one or two things in the mean time are fine; as well, it can be something from the past before you found yourself in the "rut" you are in now. If your "list" contains good things from the past before the "rut", then those are exactly the first things/character traits you need to revisit to get yourself to a better place now.

Know that optimism can be improved. Watch how kids problem solve; it's not to say that their solution works every time, but focus on the optimism in their spirits, their creative thinking, and their determination. That "child" was you once too, so this concept of optimism isn't something you have to create brand new out of thin air; it's just a matter of re-discovering what's already in you. It's important to know that things are still possible to turn out "right", or "right when you need it most", even if there are a string of things that are knocking you down currently. Having optimism is powerful, and it is a re-attainable attitude.

Find the positive in you, your past, present, and future. Also go to Chapter 8 – Stress Management –Relief: "Don't Lose Yourself".

3. Nutrition

Don't go on restrictive "fad diets"
"Fad Diets" that significantly limits what you can eat or how much you can eat will affect the hormones in your body, and this includes your mood hormones. *Disclaimer: this does not apply if you have been ordered by a doctor to be on a specific diet for health reasons.*

Increase tryptophan rich foods
Tryptophan is an amino acid found naturally in the foods that we eat. Tryptophan increases serotonin in the brain. Serotonin is the natural compound that promotes feelings of well-being and relaxation. A serotonin deficiency can result in depression, sleep disturbances, (which adds to depression), anxiety, and a propensity to overeat.

Tryptophan rich food: (healthiest foods easily available, and listed from highest to least)
Chicken, Soybeans, Turkey, Tuna, Lamb, Salmon, Halibut, Shrimp, Cod, and Sardines.

Take fish-oil supplements and eat plenty of fish

Fish oil is known to help produce the hormone Serotonin, (see paragraph above to recall information on Tryptophan and Serotonin).

4. Don't Under Sleep (Don't Over Sleep)

With a new baby, to not under sleep is easier said than done I know, but find somehow to increase sleep, (even if still not to the "proper" amount you need), and be consistent. Also don't over-sleep because it increases depressive symptoms. The quality of sleep you are getting is also important, so if you are sleeping around 7 – 8 hours a night but still don't feel refreshed, you are probably not getting quality sleep.

Sleep is a big part of depression and stress management. Please refer back to Chapter 8 – Stress Management - "ZZZZZ's Do Important Things", so you can consistently apply a few suggestions with improving your sleep.

5. Stress Management

Stress management is a big part of depression management. Please refer back to Chapter 8 – Stress Management - Relief, for a few suggestions you can consistently apply to your daily life.

6. Socialize

You many not feel like talking to anyone, but once you get going, the barrier will come down. With depression, it's easy to rationalize "why" that social gathering or one-on-one with a friend "can't" or "shouldn't" happen; so as with what I said at the beginning of this chapter, you need to make it a **good habit**, and schedule regular phone calls to friends, and face-to-face outings every few weeks. It does help, and you deserve it.

For this to consistently work, it's very important to find people that you truly have shared interests with outside of being Moms; even if this ends up only a couple key people, that's plenty enough. Talk about things besides only "mothering", and even though some of it will end up as a "vent session", definitely always include conversations that are light, positive, and about you guys as individuals. All Moms need this, so it won't be one sided, and you will be doing something your friend probably needs also.

Other Optional Treatments: (not mentioned in the "6 Things")

1. St Johns Worth: An herbal supplement popular in Europe for decades, to help treat depression. There are mixed studies saying it really works biologically, and some saying it just has a placebo effect. Taken in the appropriate dosages, it is safe for majority of people without any negative side effects.

2. Over-the-counter 5-HTP supplements: 5-HTP is made from tryptophan, and it helps the body make serotonin. Having low serotonin levels are known factors for causing mood issues. Low levels of tryptophan are most common with people who are depressed. It's important to ask your doctor about 5-HTP, to find out if you have low levels of serotonin or contradictions with taking 5-HTP.

***Important Note for both St. Johns Worth and 5-HTP*:** There is conflict to using either one of these drugs while on an anti-depressant; taking any of these drugs and an anti-depressant may cause you to have too much serotonin, (serotonin toxicity). Because 5-HTP has not been thoroughly studied in higher end clinical settings, possible side effects and interactions with other drugs are not well known.

Refer back to the section above to first try foods as a way of increasing tryptophan, rather than going straight to taking 5-HTP.

---

* If your are having a hard time managing depression, and it is getting in the way of a positively productive "life", or if you are managing "life" productively, but it is getting "too tiring" to manage it, there are places you can turn to for help. *

Where you can turn to for help:

Postpartum Support International

Phone: (805) 967-7636
Website: www.postpartum.net

Postpartum Support International offers information and support not only to women who are coping with postpartum depression and anxiety after childbirth, but also to their families. The Web site also includes the "Mills Depression", and "Anxiety Symptom-Feeling Checklist", for evaluating your symptoms.

(see more options on the next page)

....

PPD MOMS
1-800-PPD-Moms (1-800-773-6667)

PPD MOMS is a volunteer-led organization providing support services to women and their families struggling with the effects of postpartum depression (PPD), or related mood disorders.

They provide:
Telephone support
Peer support groups (*free - however a donation for the foundation is welcome*).
Referrals to professionals
Public education
Awareness and advocacy

....

www.PostPartumStress.com/books

Postpartum depression related books

....

www.DBSAlliance.org

Web site for depression. Support groups throughout the United States. Clinician referrals. Many great articles about recovery options, recovery steps, wellness, and much more.

....

www.store.samhsa.gov/mhlocator

Directory of mental health services by state and location

....

Could it be Postpartum Psychosis?

Postpartum psychosis is the most extreme form of postpartum mood disorders, and it is also the most rare.

It is usually described as a period when a woman loses touch with reality, has delusional thoughts, and the disorder occurs in women who have recently given birth.

Women with a personal or family history of psychosis, bipolar disorder, or schizophrenia, have an increased risk of developing post-partum psychosis.

Onset of symptoms can occur at anytime within the first 3 months after giving birth, but usually symptoms develop within the first 2 to 3 weeks after delivery.

Postpartum psychosis affects between one to two women per 1,000 women who have given birth; this is very low at .01 - .02%.

It is believed that fewer than 20% of Mothers with this disorder, who realize something is wrong, will actually seek help. Women who do receive proper treatment often respond well, (experiencing postpartum depression on the way to fully recovering).

Without treatment, postpartum psychosis can lead to tragic consequences. It is estimated that postpartum psychosis has a 5% suicide rate, and a 4% infanticide rate.

If you may be suffering from postpartum psychosis, it is important for you to understand that this is not your "fault", and you can't simply "will" it away; you need to do more. PLEASE seek help immediately. Your family doesn't want you to suffer, you do not have to suffer unnecessarily through this, and there is help available for you.

Symptoms of Postpartum Psychosis:
(you <u>do not</u> have to experience all of these symptoms to have post-partum psychosis)

* Hallucinations (hearing or seeing things that aren't there)
* Delusions or strange beliefs
* Rapid mood swings
* Insomnia or decreased need to sleep
* Refusing to eat
* Extreme feelings of anxiety and agitation
* Periods of confusion and disorganization (delirium)

* Periods of abnormally elevated moods or energy (mania)
* Suicidal thoughts
* Thoughts of harming you baby

It is critical to get outside professional help if you are having any of the symptoms listed above, and remember, having only one of these symptoms is enough to seek help.

Treating postpartum psychosis:

Postpartum psychosis is considered to be a mental health emergency, and therefore requires immediate attention.

Please tell someone that you are having these symptoms, (your doctor, you husband, your friend).

This condition is usually treated with medications, typically anti-psychotic drugs, and sometimes anti-depressants and/or anti-anxiety drugs.

Many Moms can also benefit from psychological counseling, and support group therapy.

Where you can go for help:

Any of the **resources mentioned for postpartum depression on pages 129 – 130,** and…

www.SuicidePreventionLifeline.org
National Suicide Prevention Hotline and Website
1-800-273-8255

Please Talk To Someone You Trust Now

Chapter Ten:

Exercise and Nutrition Concepts Made Simple

Exercise And Nutrition Plans Need To Be Done Together

For well-balanced long-term positive results, it is important to pay attention to both nutrition and exercise at the same time. It is not necessary to be "perfect" with either, but it is important to be consistent and well balanced. What I mean when I say, "being consistent", is what its basic meaning implies, being dependable, and stable. When I say, "well balanced", (in regards to exercise), I mean a program consisting of almost equally strength, cardiovascular, balance/coordination, and flexibility training. When I say, "well balanced", (in regards to nutrition), I mean having an array of food groups at each meal, with dark colored vegetables mostly filling the plate, and unhealthy fats very limited in comparison.

Nutrition alone (without exercise):

Yes, you can decrease your body fat, but often times when people diet by cutting significant amount of calories, (or "yo-yo" dieting), they will lose not just fat weight, but also valuable muscle density, and nutrients. Having dense muscles speeds up your metabolism, (which means long-term body fat maintenance), keeping your body structure stronger and safer, and making your physique look/feel healthier and younger. Exercising also keeps you athletic and physically functional; you stand and move differently when you keep yourself physically fit.

For example:
Have you heard of the term "skinny fat person"? This is a thin person who is actually higher in body fat, but still "appears" thin when it comes to body measurements. The "skinny fat" person has "thinner" muscles, which makes them look and wear smaller clothing sizes, but this person is not healthy, and her body still jiggles. Being "skinny fat" does not feel, look, or is strong and healthy; when it comes down to it, it's better to be clothing sizes higher and strong, rather than being caught up in the fake, unhealthy reward of simply some measurement numbers. *This concept also applies to the scale, (more on that a little later in this chapter).*

133

Exercise also gives you other benefits that dieting alone doesn't:
* Significantly improved energy
* Better and consistent moods
* More body awareness and control
* Increased sense of accomplishment and confidence
* Added physical skills

As we age, our metabolism naturally slows down, and our body "shrinks"; we can slow down this process with exercising/lifting weights. As we age, our basic athletic abilities, (coordination, balance, flexibility, endurance), decline significantly, if we don't use and maintain these skills either.

Exercise alone (without balanced nutrition):

You can have strong muscles or be more "athletic" because you are exercising/lifting weight, but it will be covered up with excess body fat. You have probably seen what I am talking about; that strong and muscle curved person, but not much definition, and often times you will still see excess fat on the "problem areas".

Even if a body looks fit, it can still be suffering from chronic negative nutritional ailments.

A few examples:
1. There are fit individuals who still suffer from high bad cholesterol, which can lead to heart disease.
2. The fit individual who is eating too much sugar, and having multiple highs and lows through out the day with their energy and mood.
3. The fit person who doesn't eat enough fiber, often times feeling heavy, bloated, and possibly constipated.

Keep in mind also, if you are exercising regularly, you <u>need proper nutrition to support your training</u>, and help your body recover properly.

Number One Benefit For Exercise And Nutrition At The Same Time

#1 - Maintaining a consistent nutrition AND exercise plan on a regular basis <u>is what allows you to have flexibility, and not have to be "so perfect"</u> with either category.

It's a give and receive process, so if on the few occasions you deviate from the consistent norm, it will still allow you to do that without affecting your progress or maintenance.

When you see this #1 benefit to be true, you won't feel as though you are "failing" when you have the occasional "off" days, which means you will less likely fall-off track permanently.

Get Real Results From You Fitness Training

It's important for everyone to understand that <u>if you want real results from your training</u>, then you need to <u>push yourself hard 3 days a week</u>. What I mean by "push yourself hard", is that when you are training, you want to push yourself intermittently at 80-90% of your max effort, (and depending on what type of training you are doing), with brief breaks at 50% of your effort, or a brief break all together. <u>Your body needs to get out of its comfort zone if you want real results, period</u>.

Another important concept to understand is that since your body immediately starts to adapt to its stressors, (in this case exercise), you <u>need to switch up what you are doing for your hard training, so you don't plateau</u>; good news is that it's not as complicated as it sounds. It doesn't matter if you amp up the existing training you are doing to make it more challenging, (so you are continually at the 80-90% efforts that's necessary), or you switch to an entirely new type of training all together, (as long as that training requires you to be at 80-90% efforts also).

Whether it's rotating between different types of training within a week, (i.e. 5K training and strength/balance training at the gym), or you choose a type of training that allows you to get in a well-rounded workout each training session, (i.e. outdoor boot camp), the main thing is that you are getting in a full-range of fitness basics on a regular basis, (strength, cardio, functional, balance/coordination, flexibility), for true fitness for health.

Important Note: Because your body needs recovery after training very hard, it's HIGHLY recommended to not have the "hard days" back to back.

To sum up it up:

* If you only can train 3 days a week, then all 3 days needs to be done "hard".

* If you train 5 days a week, then 3 days needs to be "hard", and the other 2 days can be "easy" or "moderate", (depending on how you feel).

* If you train 7 days a week, then 3 days needs to be "hard", and the other 4 days should be split between "moderate" and "easy" days.

You get the jest...

Monitor Your Improvements

If you don't understand the different gauges of improvements, you can't accurately access if and when things need to be modified, and you can get easily discouraged. Getting discouraged will decrease your motivation. Decreased motivation makes discipline very hard to maintain. Without discipline, you will not be consistent. You need to stay consistent in order to reach your goals.

1. Don't only go by the scale:

A. At the beginning of re-starting an exercise regimen after a long hiatus, or if you are formally exercising for the first time in your life, you can't only gauge improvements by weight; you have to go by your body fat level, how your clothes are fitting, and how you are feeling and functioning.

Often times with the first month of training, (whether training properly for the first time or after a long break), and especially when strength training is included, the scale can be deceiving. Here is why. If in the first month of training you lose 3 pounds of fat, but you gained 3 pounds of muscle, the scale shows no difference, but because one pound of fat is a "larger mass" than one pound of muscle, you will still actually be "smaller", less jiggly, more tone, and can start fitting your clothes a bit better. Note: This may happen with the initial month or so of training; if the scale does not budge after that time, it is important to reassess your nutrition and exercise plan.

B. Right after having a baby, it takes weeks/months for Moms to lose the excess water retention weight gain. Don't automatically assume that the extra "puffy" you see, feel, or weigh, are all from body fat.

2. Focus on all physical aspects of improvement besides just your weight:

Focus should be placed on regaining your abdominal/core and pelvis floor muscle's posture, strength, tone, and muscle reactions; this is initially the most important priority for post pregnancy recovery, (along with postpartum depression management if it applies).

Also when training, focus on your regained athletic/functional conditioning, lessened body aches, (particularly the back and joints), and better body posture. When we were pregnant, all of those just mentioned were affected, some more negatively than others. Didn't we miss the basics of our physical abilities that we had before our bodies were "taken over" by our baby? When training, think about how great it feels to jump, lift our knees and kick, or run; basically don't take it for granted.

3. Set goals that have nothing to do with the way you look:

It helps to set a goal that has nothing to do with the way you "look". For example, sign-up to do a local 5K, and inspire a few people to join you. By having a performance goal in mind, you will train with more motivation/discipline, and have a multi-purpose focus, (especially when you have a shared goal with other people). While your focus is on performance, and being consistent to reach that performance goal, you will eventually see a "scale" and figure improvements along the way, without being obsessed with it.

Take Advantage Of Your Hormones For Post Pregnancy Recovery

Right after having your baby, you have hormones released in your body that helps with the shrinking and repairing process. <u>We hear about hormones helping shrink our uterus, but our hormones also help shrink our skin, tighten our tendons/ligaments, and our muscles too.</u>

It's critical that you start applying the Ishio Method – Post Pregnancy Rehab Key Principles TM, and the Ishio Method – Post Pregnancy Rehab Pelvic floor/Abdominal Rehab Protocol's TM immediately, because you will have the best responses and results with your efforts by applying them early on.

After getting clearance from your OBGYN, (usually between 6 – 10 weeks post partum), the sooner you start an exercise program, (based on your comfort level, and gently consistently increasing the intensity), the more your mind and body responds to getting back to pre-pregnancy shape.

As far as the skin goes, exercising helps purge the excess water weight that we carried during pregnancy, and helps decrease the extra body fat we gained; which means when there is less excess in between our skin and our muscles, we are allowing our skin to be able to shrink down to it's maximum ability. Don't forget that exercise also helps make our muscles denser, (which speeds up our metabolism to help decrease body fat), helps manage our rapidly changing mood hormones, and helps with managing sleep and stress.

If Certain Exercises You Used To Do Before Pregnancy Are Now Painful

It is your body telling you that you are starting that particular exercise, or increasing the intensity too soon; temporarily lighten up on the movements, or eliminate them all together if necessary.

<u>This pain not a cue to automatically stop exercising all together, it is just a cue to modify your exercise, or find an alternative in the mean time.</u> You want to stay on track with a consistent routine so you can get the positive results that you want and need. Your joints, ligaments, tendons, etc, need time to revert back to normal so be careful, but many Mothers have found temporary alternative exercises until they were able to re-introduce gradually what they used to do.

Important: If "everyday" movements are causing you pain, and it is difficult for you to function, seek the help of a women's health physical therapist; being in that type of physical pain is not "normal". You don't want to get progressively worse, and you don't need daily functioning to be this difficult, lowering the quality of your life. Women's health physical therapists are not a well-known option for new Moms, or even well-known to other medical professionals, (which is why most of us are not referred to them when we open up about any pelvis area issues), so I would like to take this time to inform Moms that women's health physical therapists are out there to successfully help.

When It Comes To Your Health Plan

1. Make the plan YOUR realistic plan.

Don't be so stressed that you must do what your friend, or your neighbor, or the fad you saw on TV that worked for 100 people, sway you away from what is the best for you. When you put a plan together, <u>base your plan realistically on your available schedule, location, budget, likes and dislikes</u>; if not, you are just setting yourself up for an experience that will be discouraging and negative.

2. Maintaining a reached goal is easier then the process of getting to that goal.

What I mean by this is, initially losing the 35 pounds is a tougher process than the maintaining of the weight/figure once you get there; this is encouraging information to have, so you know that <u>the initial hard work DOES get easier</u>. By getting fit and healthy through a "lifestyle" creation/change, (with its trials and errors), you <u>WILL FIND YOUR "ZONE"</u>. Your personal **"zone"** is knowing exactly what you like to eat and do for exercise <u>that works</u>, what schedule <u>works best for your life</u>, what types of training partners or environments <u>advances your motivation</u>, and where you need to "go to" in your mind to help <u>maintain discipline</u>, etc.

3. The first time you do any new exercise, it will most likely get you sore. Depending on the intensity, it will get you very sore.

Two things that needs to be understood to get you through those days:

One is, the next time you do the same movements, you will never get as sore as the first time, (as long as a long time doesn't pass with you doing the same exercise again).

Second, when you are sore, it is because that exercise caused many small muscle fiber tears in those parts of your body. Good news is that your body will immediately start repairing itself. When you are not sore any more, that means you body has healed, and those muscles are now stronger than before. There is a benefit to that mild to moderate soreness.

4. Don't just quit your plan because you didn't stick with it 100%.

While you are figuring out your personal "zone", there will need to be some tinkering done.

Also, know that you don't need to be perfect to reach your goals, AND REALLY KNOW that by quitting, you have a 0% chance of reaching your goals?

Remember as with #2, getting there is the really hard part, (rough waters), and the "maintaining" is smoother sailing.

Basically what I'm saying is, don't quit. If you feel absolutely sure you can't, then re-visit #1 in this section, and re-plan a more realistic plan for yourself.

Important Tools Available To Help With Success (sheets are in chapter 12)

"Lifestyle Log": this is <u>highly recommended</u> for those that have poor nutritional habits, (food choices, over-eating, under-eating, or having long periods go by without eating).

The Lifestyle Log is so you can get an idea of what your current nutritional, (and exercise), habits are. Log for 1 full week, review at the end of that week, and you will be able to see your habits accurately. Make notes on any necessary adjustments you need to make, <u>while continue</u> logging for at least another few months, (and longer if needed to maintain discipline).

After using the Lifestyle Log for a little while, eventually, you will be able to simply reflect on your day/week, and know if you are still "in" the nutritional and exercise plan that is part of your personal health "zone".

"Workout Check-off Sheet": this is <u>highly recommended</u> if you require more help with exercise discipline.

This is a simple one-page sheet that you simply check-off everyday on whether you did your workout as planned, (or had a scheduled day-off as planned). You can also modify/swap workouts if necessary. This one sheet tracks an entire 4-weeks worth of workouts, (that's how simple it is), and helps with holding you accountable for the plan you set for yourself, and adds to your sense of accomplishment.

You can modify the training week by week as you need, for example, if you know you will be out of town for a week, or during spring break and the kids are out of school, etc.

"Workout Plan Reference Sheet": this as a reference sheet you refer to when filling out your "Work-out Check-off Sheet" every 4-weeks.

"Top-10 Nutrition Favorites Sheet": this is a reference sheet for a quick way to recall your favorite foods and portion sizes that is based off your needs. By filling it out in the first place, it helps you reinforce at a conscious and subconscious level, what your plan is.

Chapter Eleven:

Starter Fitness Programs

Important Note: Do not start any exercise program until after you have clearance from your doctor that it is okay for you to start exercising. Please pay attention to your body, use reasonable judgment when trying any new movements/exercises, and if in doubt, skip any exercises you feel necessary.

Starter Fitness Program General Information

* The starter fitness workouts are intended to give you a good start for if you are not sure what to do, want to ease back to the training you were doing before pregnancy, or want to try something different from what you were doing before.

* All workouts start with a basic warm-up, and end with cool-down stretches that target every major muscle group.

* Each circuit level includes a mix of cardio, strength training, and plyometric exercises. All are designed to help rebuild better physical function and athleticism after pregnancy, to improve balance/coordination, and offer over-all muscle and cardiovascular system conditioning.

* There are 3 difficulty levels (program 1, 2, and 3), and 3 weekly commitment levels, (short burst, maximize, and full-throttle).

* All circuit workouts are designed so you can do them indoors at home, in the back yard, at a park, or gym. They are also designed to not need any equipment except for dumbbells. Since it's home friendly, you can do this while your kids are napping, or while they are in the same room with you.

* You can swap out any exercises with something else you've done before, (as long as it's still targeting the same purpose of what's being swapped out).

Progressing From Fitness Program 1, 2, and 3

With this "Starter Fitness Program", Program 1 is the easiest level, Program 2 is a little more challenging, and Program 3 is the most challenging.

Do not go on to Program #2 unless you are doing Program #1 correctly. Just the same, do not go onto Program #3, unless you are able to do Program #2 correctly.

Rushing to do the more difficult exercises will not get you into better shape faster if you are not ready for them. Doing the exercises incorrectly defeats the intended purpose, it can get you injured, as well, without proper posture with the easier exercises, advancing to the next level will most likely only have your posture worsen.

Weekly Commitment

"Short Burst" – 3 days a week – 3 circuits each session
"Full Throttle" – 4 days a week – 3 circuits each session
"Maximize" – 5 days a week – 3 circuit days/3 circuits per session AND 2 days Running
intervals.

For the "short burst" and "full-throttle" commitment levels, you can swap out a circuit day with a Running Interval day.

Standard Warm-up Routine And Cool-down Stretches

It's important not to skip the few minutes of warm-ups before doing the circuit or interval running, or skip doing the cool-down stretches afterwards. The warm-ups will get your body loosened up and ready for more dynamic movements, while lessening injury. The stretches will help cool-down your body, help your body recover faster, and with more flexibility, it helps prevent injuries, and improve over-all body functions.

Later in this chapter, there will be detailed directions, with photos, for both the Standard Warm-up routine, and the standard Cool-down Stretches.

Important Tools Available To Help With Success (sheets are in chapter 12)

"Workout Check-off Sheet": this is <u>highly recommended</u> if you require more help with exercise discipline.

This is a simple one-page sheet that you simply check-off everyday on whether you did your workout as planned, (or had a scheduled day-off as planned). You can also modify/swap workouts if necessary. This one sheet tracks an entire 4-weeks worth of workouts, (that's how simple it is), and helps with holding you accountable for the plan you set for yourself, and adds to your sense of accomplishment.

You can modify the training week by week as you need, for example, if you know you will be out of town for a week, or during spring break and the kids are out of school, etc.

"Workout Plan Reference Sheet": this as a reference sheet you refer to when filling out your "Work-out Check-off Sheet" every 4-weeks.

Standard Warm-up Routine *(for all circuit programs)*

Warm-up List:
Neck Circles
Hip Circles
Knee Circles
Ankle Circles
Helicopter Spins
Shoulder/Arm Circles
Kick Checks
Chest Pumps
Feet Shuffle
Jumping Jacks

....

<u>Neck Circles:</u>
Start by looking down towards one side of your body, and then circle your head back while your face looks up towards looking the sky, then down to the other side.

Do 10 rotations circling to the left, and then 10 rotations circling to the right.

(see photos on the next page)

143

Neck Circles

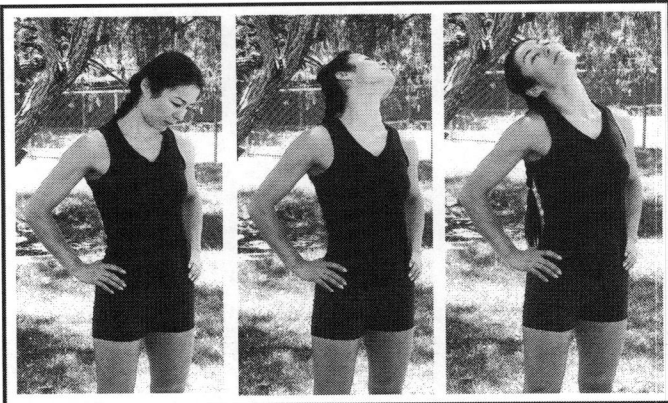

....

Hip Circles:

Place your hands on your hips. Leading with your hips, start moving them to one side, and "make" a big circle with your hips until you end up at the starting point again.

Do 10 big rotations to the left, then 10 rotations to the right.

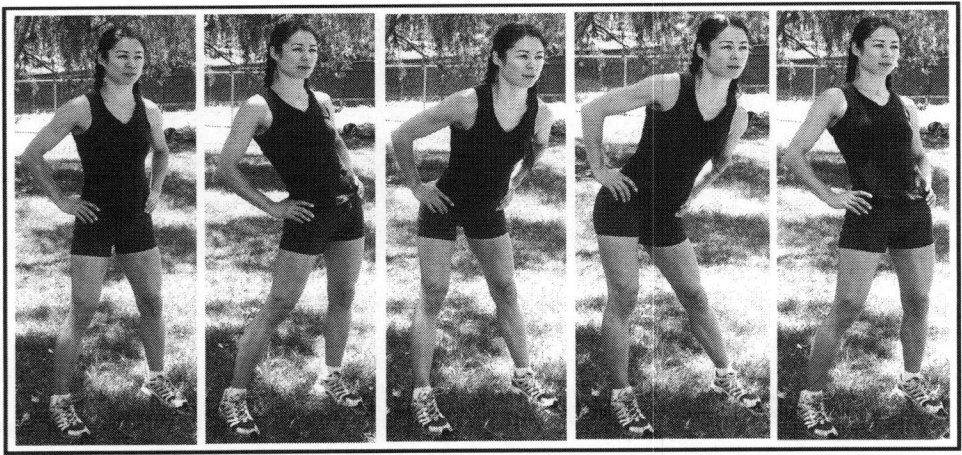

....

Knee Circles:

Bend your knees AS you sit your butt backwards, (so that way you are using your thighs to hold up your body, and not putting most of the pressure on your knees). Lightly place the heels of your palms above your knees. Leading with your knees, carefully start moving them to one side, and "make" a small circle with your knees, until you end up at the starting point again.

Do 10 small rotations to the left, then 10 rotations to the right.

(see photos on the next page)

Knee Circles

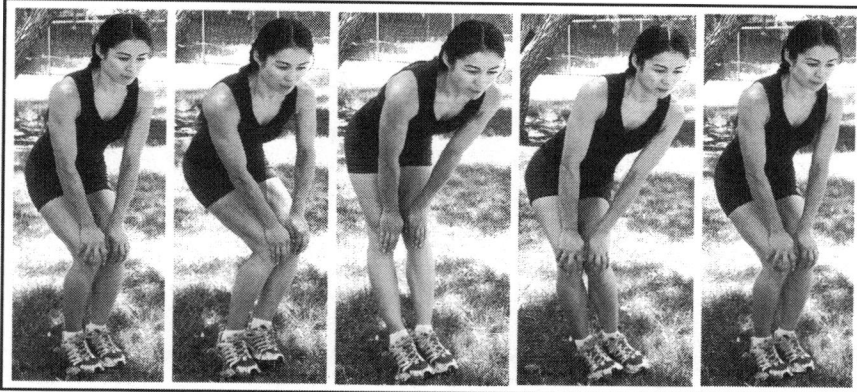

....

Ankle Circles:

Place your hands on your hips. Lightly place one foot onto the tip of its toes. Rotate the heel of your foot in a small "circle", allowing your ankle to rotate also.

Do this 5 count to the left, and then 5 count to the right, then switch foot and repeat.

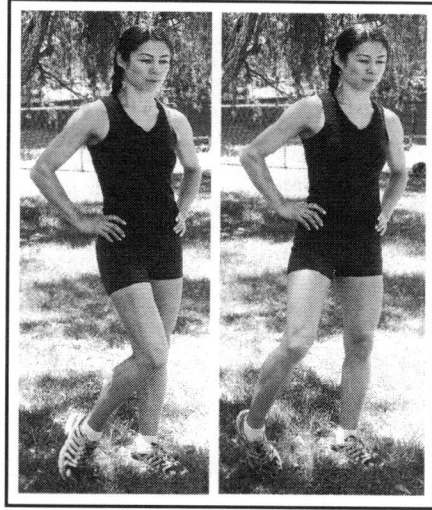

....

Helicopter Spins:

Stand with good posture, and your feet hip width apart. Open your arms out to your sides, then swing to one side as far as you can turn, then swing to the other side as far as you can turn.

Swinging to the left, and then to right is one count; do 10 counts.

(see photos on the next page)

Helicopter Spins

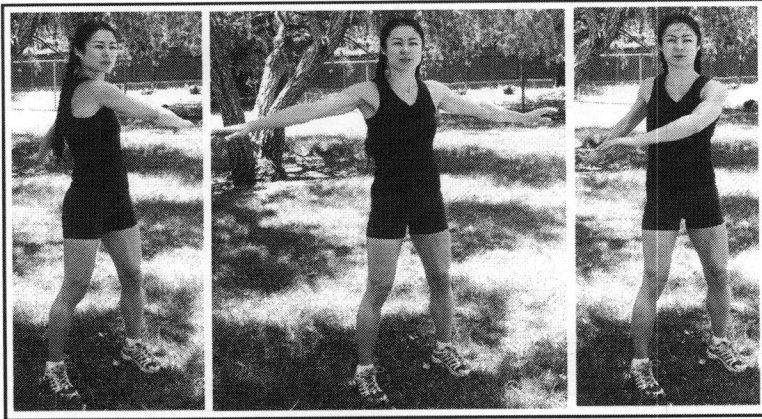

....

Shoulder/Arm Circles:

Stand with good posture. Start with arms down at your sides. Swing them through a full circle, starting with going forward in front of your body, and continuing through behind your body.

Do 10 count forward circles, and then 10 count backwards circles.

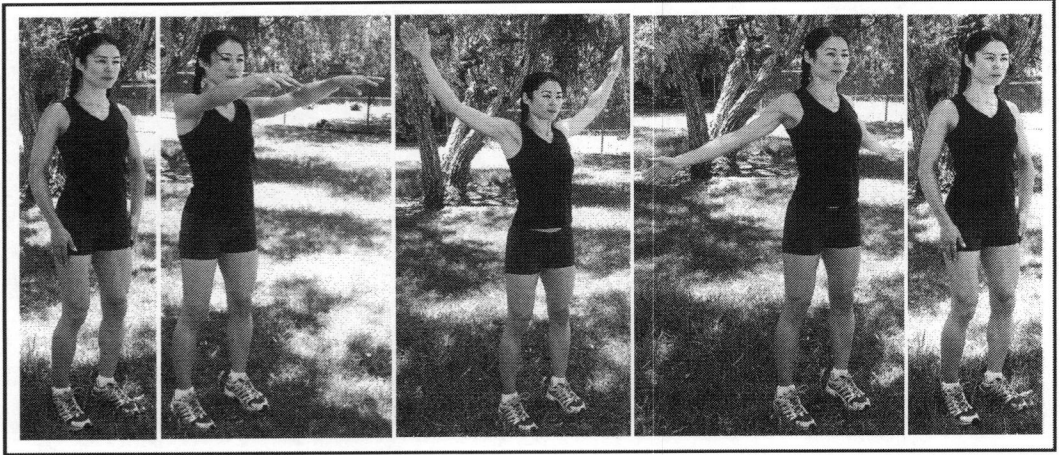

....

<u>Kick Checks</u>:

Stand with one leg in front of the other, and lift your fists up to shoulder level in front of you. Now lift your back knee up as high as you can, in front of you. Once in front, rotate that knee out to the side of your body as much as possible, (while keeping your knees up high). After your knee has rotated out to the sides of your body as far as it can go, bring the knee down and place your feet back to the starting position.

Do this rotation for 10 count with your left leg, then do the same thing for your right leg.

146

Kick Checks

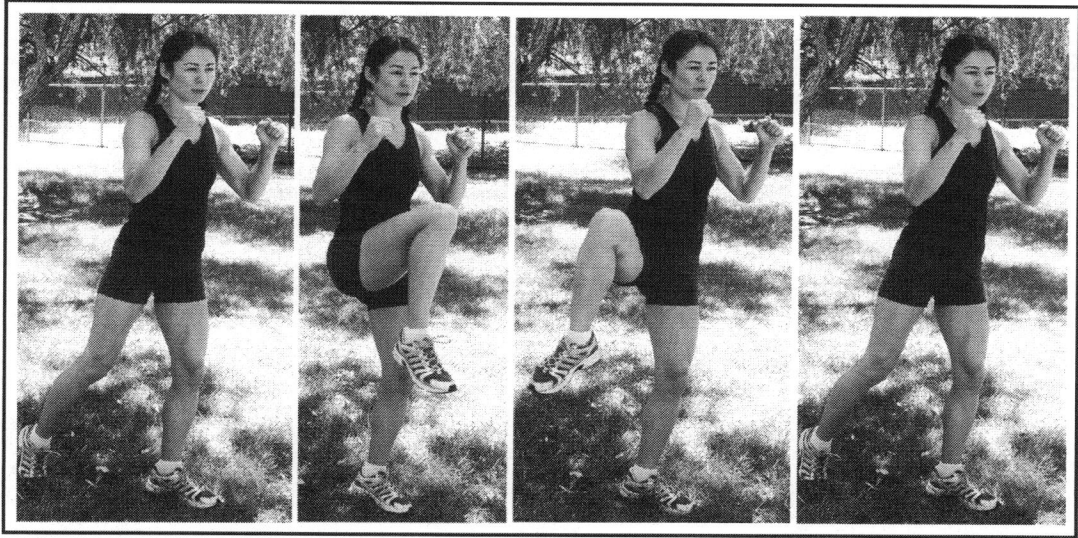

....

Chest Pumps:

Start with your arms extended in front of you; this is your starting position. Now open your arms out to your sides, lifting your chest open, while turning your hands over so your palms are facing the sky.

Allow your torso to slightly lean back as you are opening up your arms, but remember you must pull-in your abdominal muscles when leaning back, (or else you will be popping out your abdominal muscles).

Do 10 chest pumps.

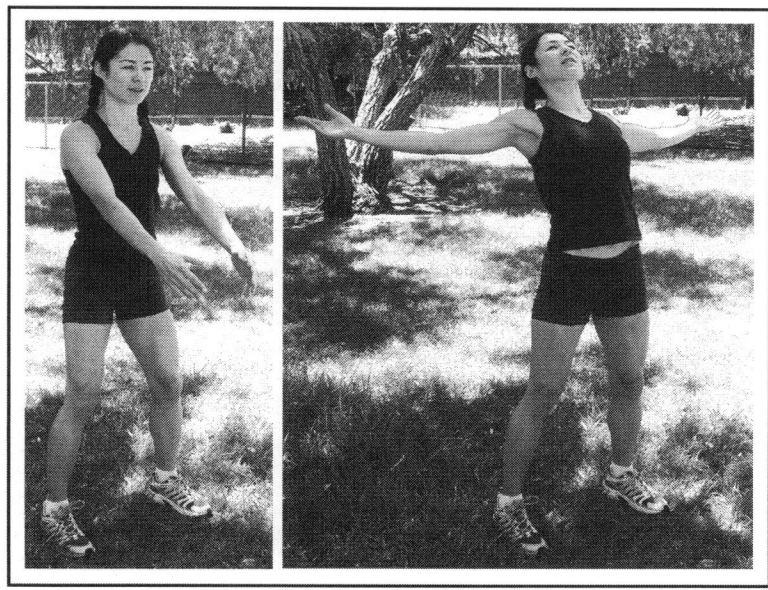

Feet Shuffle:

Stand with one leg in front, and one leg in back. Keep your arms bent, and relaxed. Shift your weight back until more than 95% of your weight is on your back leg. Now using the back leg, push off, creating a significant and controlled <u>hop forward</u>, ending with more than 95% of your weight now on your front leg. <u>Immediately</u>, push off the front leg, until your weight is back 95% onto your back leg. <u>You want the forwards and backwards "hops" to be quick and consecutive</u>.

Do this 20 count back and forth, left leg lead, and then 20 count back and forth, right leg lead.

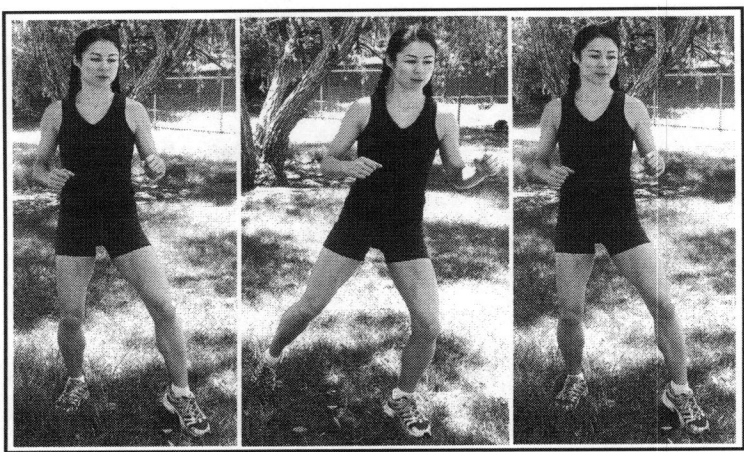

Jumping Jacks:

Start by standing with "good posture", feet shoulder width apart, and hands down at the sides of your body. Now "pop" open your feet, WHILE you raise your hands out to the sides until they touch each other above your head. Once your hands touch, immediately hop your feet back "in" WHILE you lower your arms back to the starting position.   Do 5 sets of 10 count.

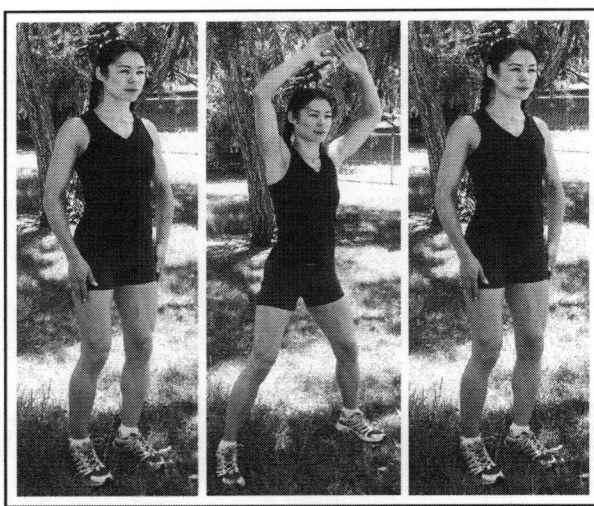

****

<u>Standard Cool-down Stretches</u> (AFTER working out)
(for all 3 circuit or running interval programs)

Stretching List:

Calve
IT Band (leg tendon)
Hamstring - Position 2 (hips pushed backwards)
Quadriceps (Quads)
Triceps (back of arm)
Chest

....

<u>Calve Stretch:</u>
Find a wall, tree, sign pole, etc. While keeping your heel on the ground and as close to the fixed object as possible, place the top half of your foot onto the fixed object. Now, move your hips, (see middle photo), and not your torso, (see last photo), towards the fixed object.

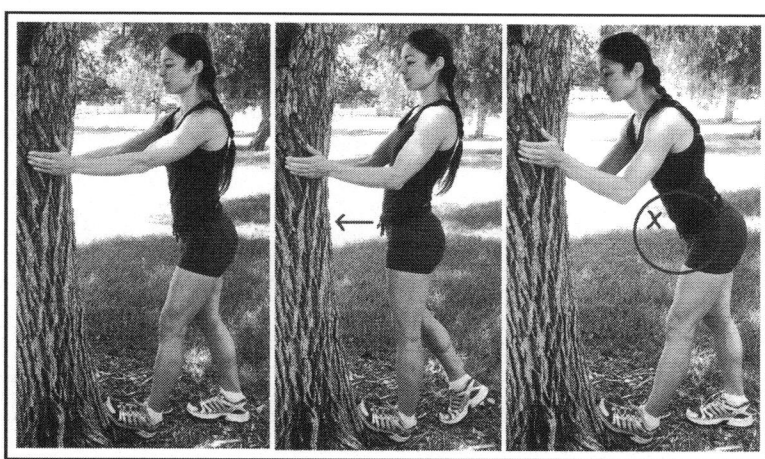

....

IT Band Stretch (leg tendon)

For a refresher: on details with foot position and body alignment, please <u>refer back to Chapter 6 – Balansu Therapy тм, on pages 84 and 85</u>.

(see photos on the next page)

See how the standing foot is forward   *The side with the leg up, ROLL that hip down.*

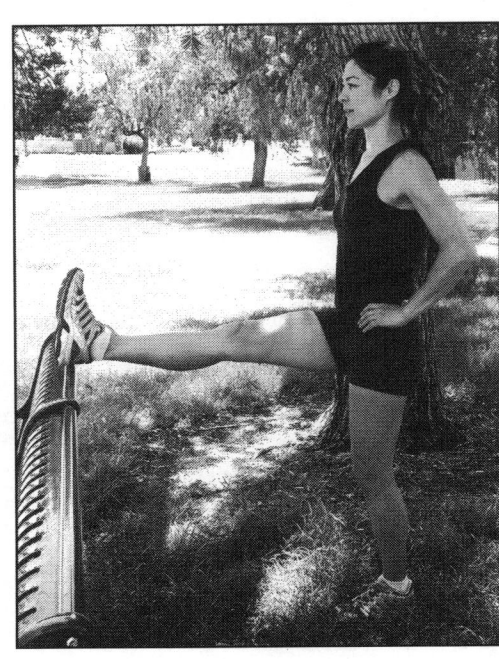
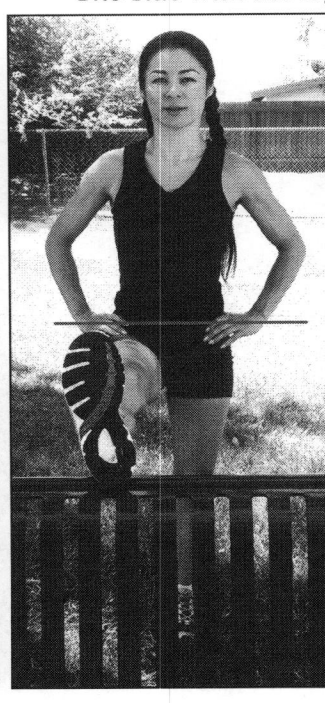
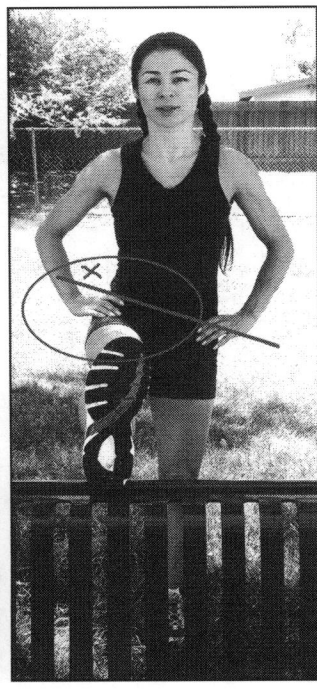

Hamstring Stretch - Position 2 (hips pushed backwards)

For a refresher: *on details with foot position and body alignment, please* <u>*refer back to Chapter 6 – Balansu Therapy* TM*, pages 83 and 84*</u>.

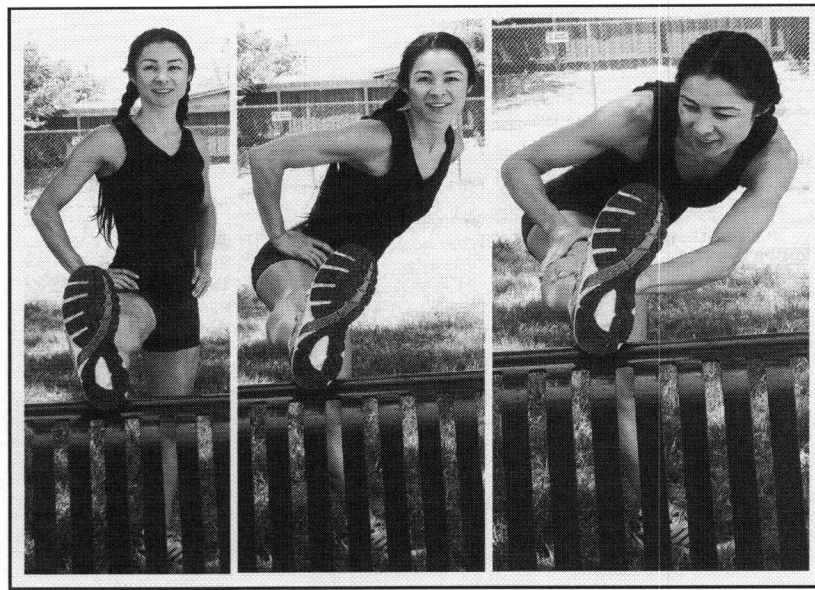

Quadriceps Stretch (**Quads**):

Hold onto a fixed object with one hand for balance. Using the hand that's on the same side as the leg you are going to stretch, grab the instep and hold. Now gently pull that leg backwards until that knee is behind the standing leg's knee. To maximize the length of the quad stretch, go into the "Ideal Core Box Posture", (as we talked about on page 15), without letting your bent knee move in front of your "standing leg's" knee. *(see the pelvis difference between both photos)*

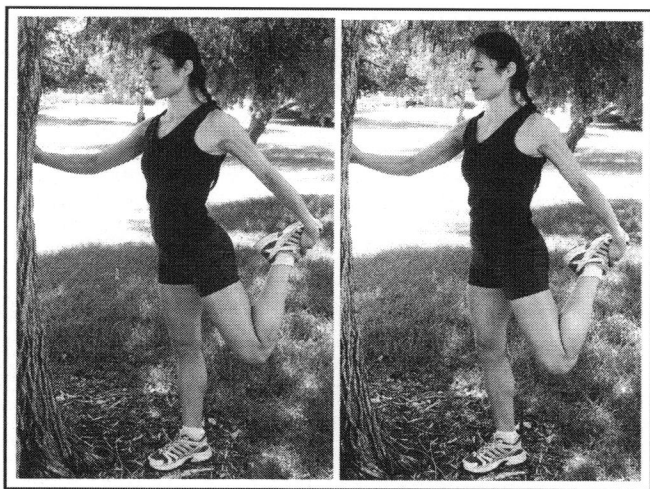

Triceps Stretch:

Lift one arm up towards the ceiling. Now bend that arm so its hand lays by your shoulder at your back. Put your other hand over your head and grab the bent arm's elbow. Now gently pull the bent elbow up towards the ceiling, <u>while simultaneously</u> drawing the elbow back behind you.

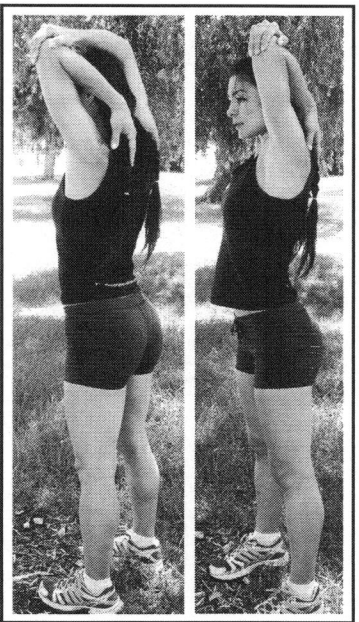

Chest Stretch: (this stretch also helps stretch the biceps)

For a refresher: on details with foot position and body alignment, please <u>refer back to Chapter 6 – Balansu Therapy TM on page 65</u>.

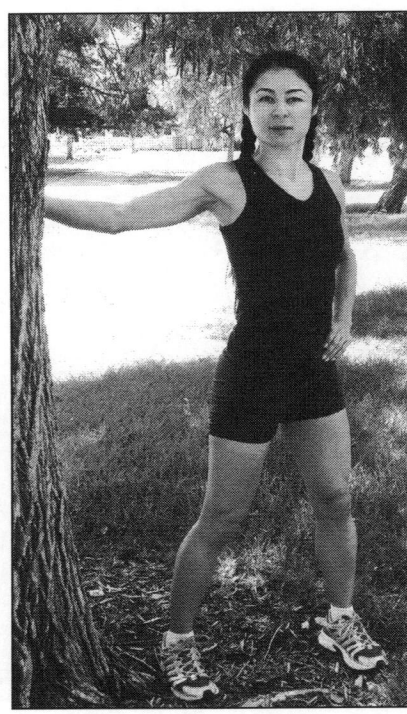 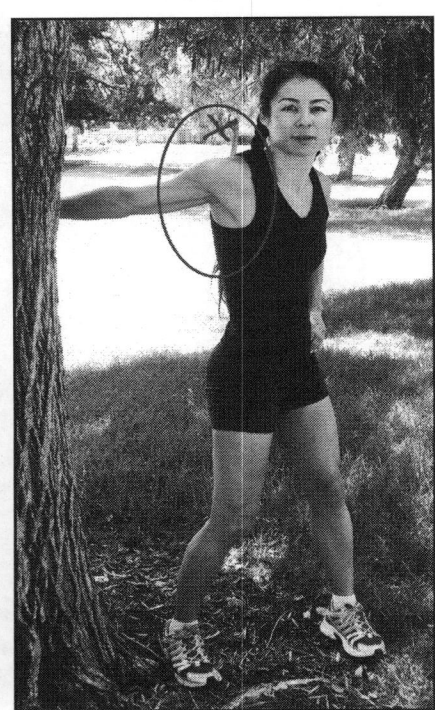

****

<u>Important Reminder While Exercising:</u>

Ishio Method – Post Pregnancy Abdominal and Pelvis Floor Rehab Key Principles TM
(Core Posture TM, Surge Posture TM, Set Posture TM, Breathe Posture TM)

<u>When doing these "Postures" while exercising, you WILL BE AMPLIFYING the rehabilitation of your abdominal and pelvis floor muscles, the entire time.</u>

****

****

Starter Program Level #1

<u>Standard warm-up</u>: for reminder, refer back to earlier in this chapter.

Circuit:

Regular Squats (own body weight)
Half and Half Planks (on forearm)
Butt Kicks
Shoulder Dumbbell Fly (Bent arm)
Fast High knees (marching or jogging it)
Bicep curls
Dumbbell Fly for the Upper back (seated)
Slides (feet only)
Triceps kickback

<u>Standard stretches</u>: for reminder, refer back to earlier in this chapter.

Ishio Method <u>Pelvic Floor Rehab</u> Protocol ᴛᴍ: refer to Ch3 and Ch12, (for the check-off sheets).
Ishio Method <u>Abdominal Rehab</u> Protocol ᴛᴍ: refer to Ch4 and Ch12, (for the check-off sheets).

....

<u>Regular Squats</u>:

Stand with feet farther than shoulder width apart. <u>The first movement you want to concentrate on is with sticking your butt backwards AS YOU start bending your knees</u>; this will prevent your knees from leading the way, and going past your toes, taking all the weight.

As your butt is leading the way while moving downwards, keep bending your knees more, until there is a 90degree angle at your knees. *Note: make sure your knees aren't caving in towards each other, and they are facing the direction that your toes are facing. Also allow your upper body to tilt forward as your butt moves backwards, while keeping your shoulders pulled back, torso straight, and abdominals pulled-in.*

Do 10 repetitions.

(see photos on the next page)

153

Squat

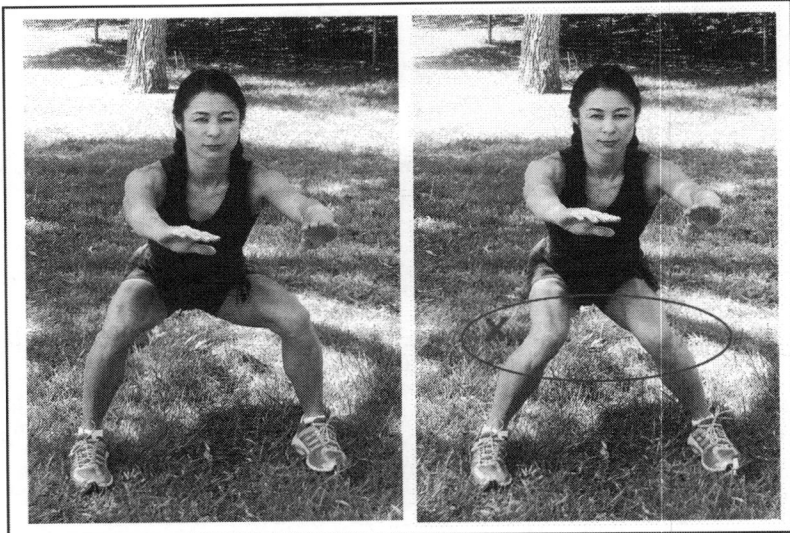

Notice how the knees don't cave in, the 90degree angle at the knees, and the torso tall while tilting forward.

Important Reminder: You must keep your knees from going over your toes, (that's what the "leading with your butt backwards" helps with). <u>JUST AS IMPOTANT</u>, make sure your knees are pointing in the direction that your toes are pointing, (no "caving in" knees).

....

Half and Half Planks (on forearm): remember, this is <u>part of your abs rehab protocol.</u>

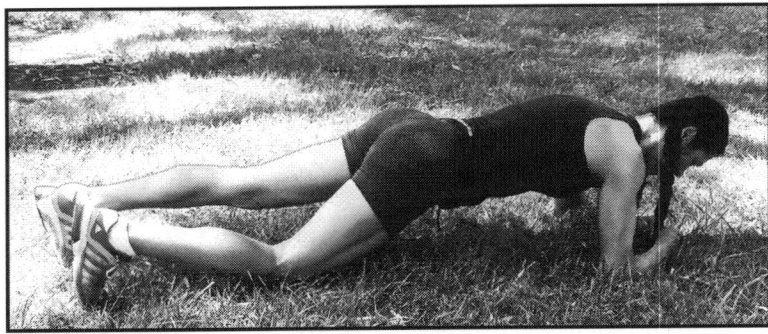

For a refresher: *please <u>refer back to Chapter 4 – Ishio Method – Abdominal Rehab Protocol ™ on page 45</u>.*

....

<u>**Butt Kicks:**</u>

You will be moving forward as you do these. Do a very light easy jog forward, then start kicking your heels up and under your butt as you continue moving forward. *Note: It's not simply slapping the back of your butt with your heels; you want to "tuck" your heels under your butt, which means your knees will have to come up slightly as you do this.* Your arms should be moving with elbows bent, with forwards and backwards motion, like you are running.

Do 30 repetitions (15 on each side).

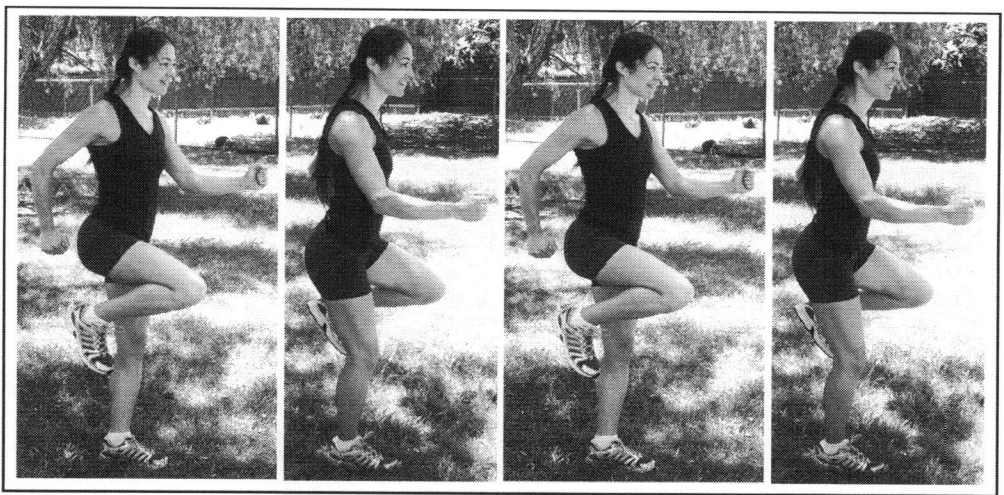

....

Shoulder Dumbbell Fly: (bent arm)

Do a body check and make sure you have "good posture", (upper body, core, and feet). Bend your elbows to about a 90degree angle. <u>While maintaining the 90degree angle the entire time, lift your elbows up, then back down.</u> *Note: Have the dumbbells in your hands be parallel with your biceps when your weights are at the top position.* Also, when you have the weights lowered back down to the starting position, don't relax your arms before lifting the weights once again; you want to keep your arms tight the entire time, so you aren't resting during a set.

Do 10 repetitions.

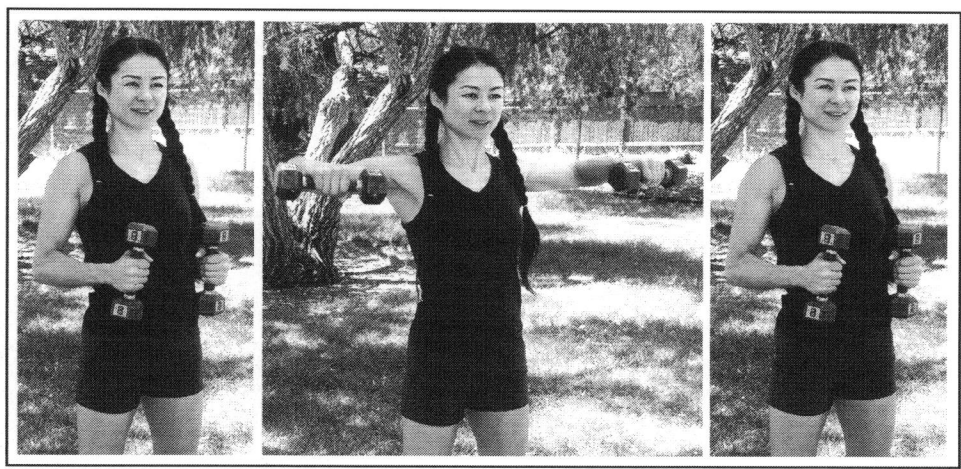

Fast High Knees:

You will be moving forward as you do these. Alternate lifting your left and right knees up and down quickly, as high as they can go, while keeping your torso tall, (no leaning backwards). Keep your abs pulled-in at all times. Your arms should be moving with elbows bent, with forwards and backwards motion like a runner. *Note: for this exercise, you should be concentrating on the knees going up and down quickly, rather than the distance you are moving forward.*

Do 20 repetitions, (10 on each side).

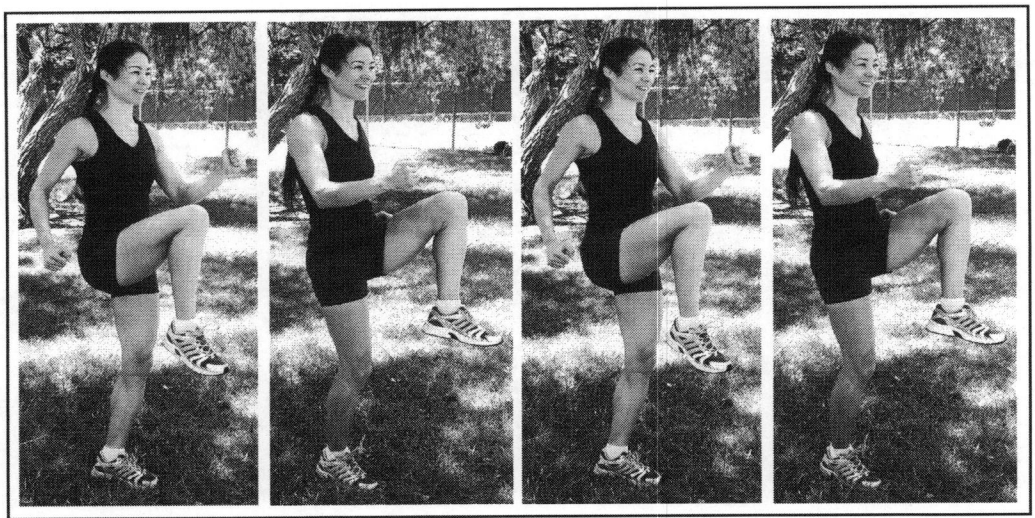

Bicep Curls:

Stand shoulder width apart, with "good posture". Place your elbows firmly down to your sides, and do not move them during the exercise. Lift the weights up and down.

Important Note: *when lifting the weights up, don't go all the way up until the weights are laying right next to your shoulders; keep the weights a slight distance away, so you are not "resting" at the top. As well, when you have the weights down at the bottom, don't allow your arms to relax; keep your muscles tight the entire time, because again, you don't want your arms to be "resting" in the middle of a set.*

Do 10 repetitions.

(See photos on the next page)

Bicep Curls

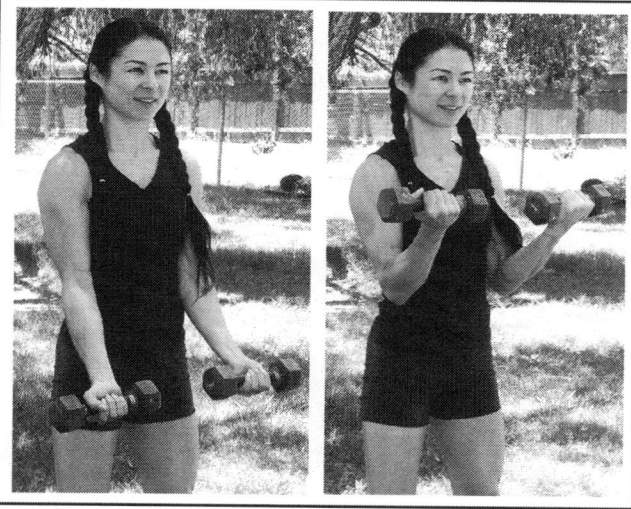

Note: Many women tend to lift too light of weights with weight training. For example, with this exercise, instead of limiting yourself with staying at 5lbs, eventually lift with 8 or 10lbs. The very vast majority of women won't get "bigger"; you will just get stronger and denser, (which is what you want).

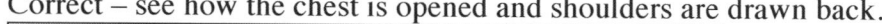

Dumbbell Fly for the Upper Back: (seated)

Sit on a chair with you torso tall, your feet under you, with your heels up. While keeping your torso tall, lean forward, <u>while</u> you keep your chest open, and shoulder blades drawn back. *Note: don't "hunch" forward, allowing your chest to collapse.* Now lift your dumbbells <u>as you continue</u> opening up your chest, and drawing your shoulder blades back some more. Once your weights are at the top, hold for half a second, <u>and with control</u>, lower your arms. *Note: once your weights are at the bottom, don't relax your arms; keep them tight so aren't "resting" them during the set.*

Do 10 repetitions.

Correct – see how the chest is opened and shoulders are drawn back.

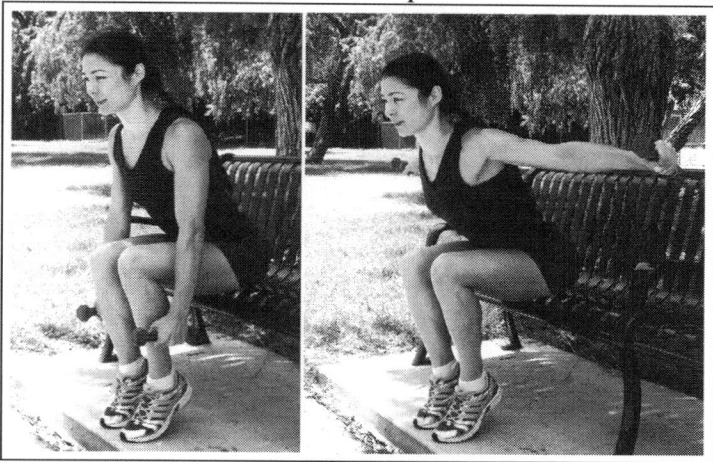

Incorrect – see how the chest is collapsed and shoulders forward

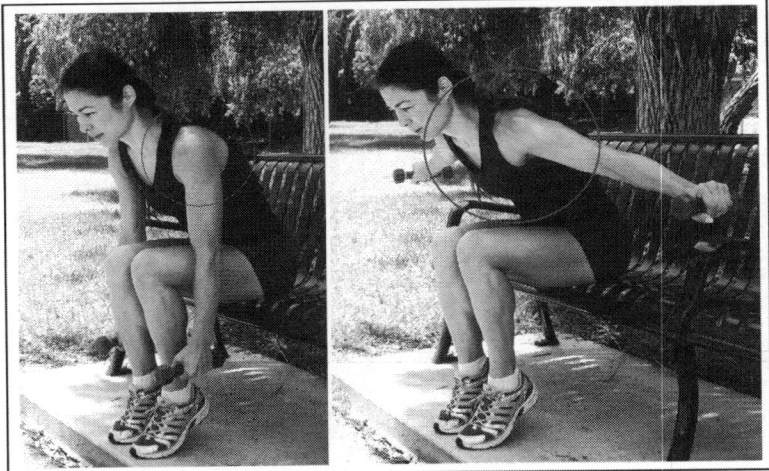

Slides:

This is an exercise that has continuous motion going sideways. Pick a direction that you will start with. Start with your feet together, and use the "back" leg, (leg opposite of the direction you are going), and push off and get some airtime going sideways with your body. As soon as your "front" foot lands, immediately bring the "back" trailing leg in, and use that same "back" leg to launch yourself again. This will be done in continuous motion, so you should never be on both legs at the same time for more than a fraction of a second.

Do 10 count push-offs going one direction, then <u>without turning yourself around</u>, (so you can get the "opposite side" of your body), repeat the same thing towards the direction you just came from.

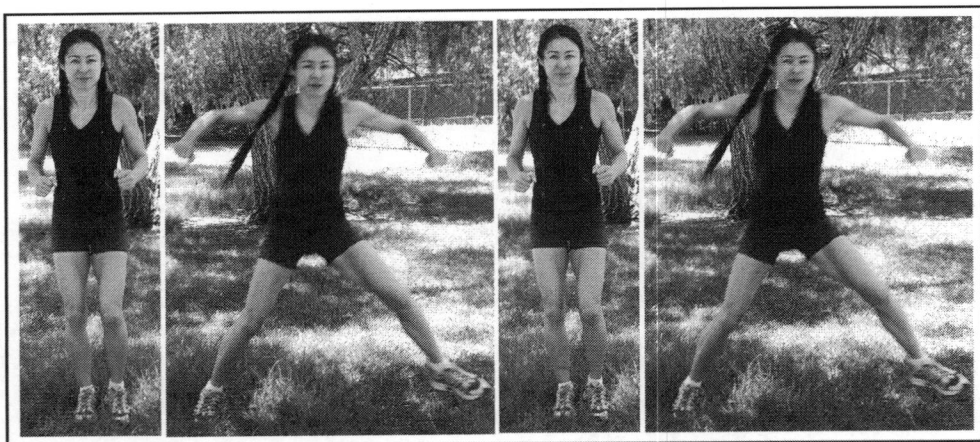

Triceps Kickbacks:

Use the back of a park bench, a chair, or something of that height. With the arm that isn't holding the dumbbell, use that arm to hold yourself up on the bench; don't lock the elbow, so you can work out that arm's muscles too. Extend straight behind you, (without locking your knee), the leg that's on the same side as the arm that's holding the weight. *Note: for balance, make sure your feet are shoulder width apart, as in, don't stand like you are on a balance beam.*

Now lift the elbow of the arm that is holding the dumbbell. Make sure you are keeping that arm tight against the side of your body.

Important Note: *make sure you aren't shrugging your shoulders; you don't want that to be your standing posture, so you don't want to reinforce that type of posture while exercising.*

While keeping your arm and elbow in this starting position the entire time, with control, extend your forearm to "open and close". *Note: If you want the exercise to be more challenging, every time you extend your arm "open", squeeze your arm against the side of your body.*

Do 10 repetitions on each arm.

Correct   Incorrect

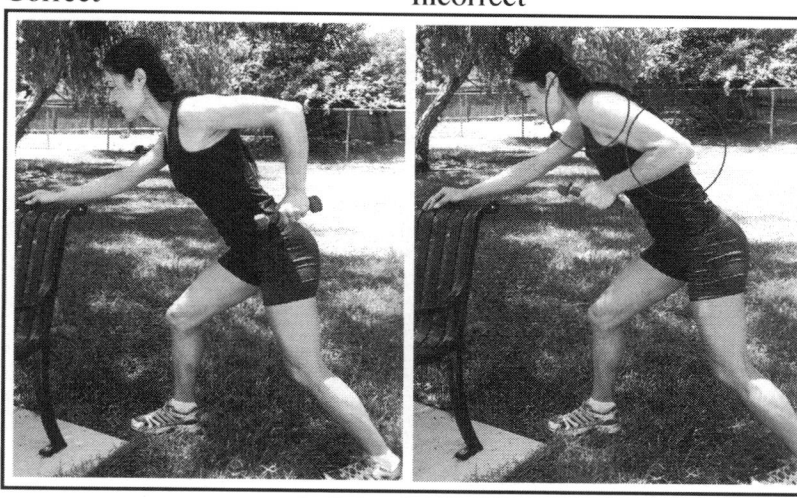

Correct   Incorrect

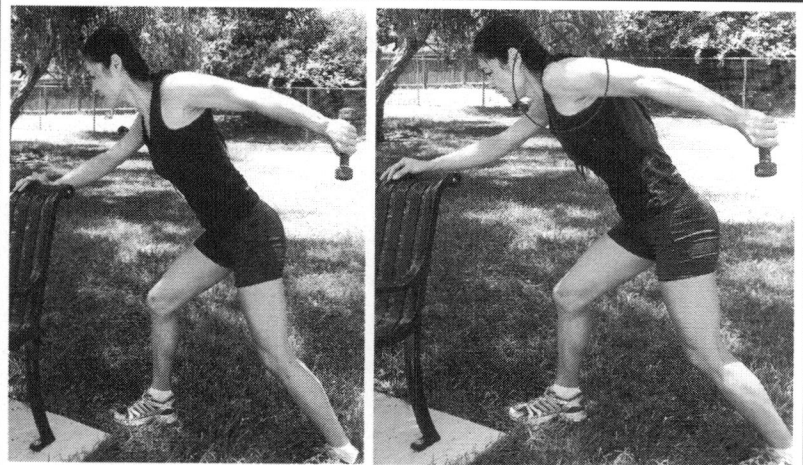

....

"Full-throttle" Program (level 1)
(running intervals for additional 2 days of training)

* These can be done at a park, or around the neighborhood, and with a baby jogger, or a training partner *

Warm-up:
walk/jog mix - 10 minutes

Intervals:
"Speed Play" – 10 - 15 minutes

Directions:
1. (Use a stopwatch). Simply start the stopwatch.
2. Run at 75 - 80% max effort for as long as you can; approximately 20 seconds to 1 minute.
3. After the 75 - 80% run, walk fast, or a very easy jog for a recovery…approximately 1 minute.
4. Repeat steps #2 and #3 until your stopwatch reaches 10 - 15 minutes.

Cool-down:
walk/jog mix - 5 minutes.

Stretches: standard stretches as noted.

****

Starter Program Level #2:

Standard Warm-up: for reminder, refer back to earlier in this chapter.

Circuit:
Jump Squats
Upper body Plank (on forearms)
Kick-outs
Dumbbell Jabs
Double Leg Hops
Biceps Curl with Lift
Dumbbell Back and Lift
Slides with Twists
Triceps Over-head press

Standard Stretches: for reminder, refer back to earlier in this chapter.

Ishio Method Pelvic Floor Rehab Protocol ™: refer to Ch3 and Ch12, (for the check-off sheets).
Ishio Method Abdominal Rehab Protocol ™: refer to Ch4 and Ch12, (for the check-off sheets).

Jump Squats:

Jump squats are just like the squats that are part of Starter Program # 1, except you will add a jump as you lift your body from the squat.

Stand with feet farther than shoulder width apart. Go into a squat and touch the ground.

Reminder: the first movement you want to concentrate on is with sticking your butt backwards AS YOU start bending your knees. Go down to a 90degree angle at your knees, and make sure your knees aren't caving in towards each. Also allow a tall upper body to tilt forward as your butt moves backwards.

As you come up, continue into a jump with arms extended above you towards the sky, and as you are landing, immediately go into another squat to start the next rep right after this rep.

IMPORTANT: as you land, and at the first hint of touching the ground, you MUST stick out your butt backwards AS you bend your knees, so you can make sure that you are using your thighs to take the force of the landing, and NOT your knees. Also make sure that when you are at the "squat position", that you are actually in a squat, and not just touching the ground with your hands, but still having your butt in the air.

Start with 3 consecutive Jump Squats in a row, then a short break, for another set of 3. Your goal is to do 10 consecutive Jump Squats in a row.

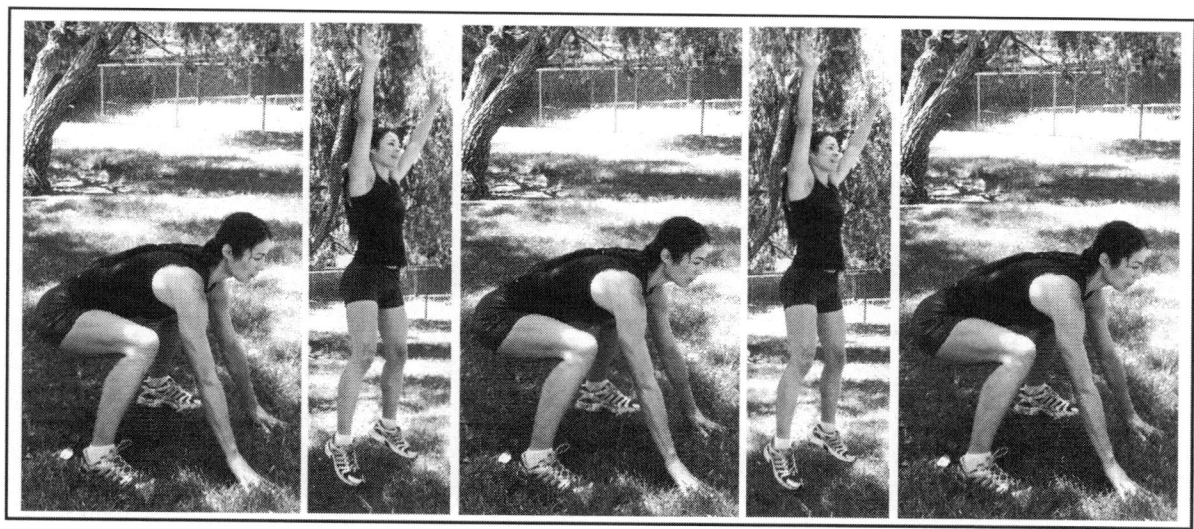

Upper body Plank (on forearms): remember, this is part of your abs rehab protocol.

For a refresher with "Planks": please refer back to Chapter 4 – Ishio Method – Abdomianl Rehab Protocol on page 53.

(see photo on the next page)

Upper-body Plank

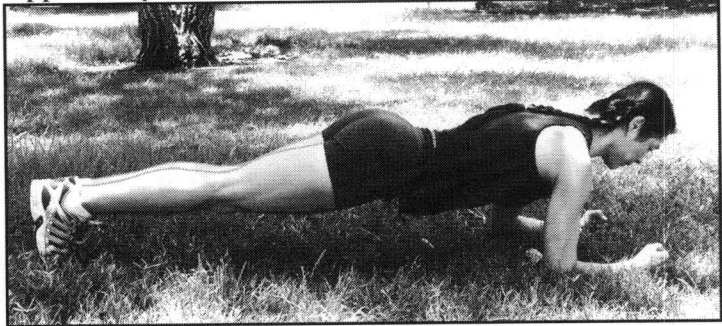

....

Kick-outs:

For this exercise, you will be continuously moving forward. Start with one leg in front of the other. Lift your back knee up and kick out your foot, (leading with the heal). Once that foot hits the ground, lift your other knee up, (which now is the "back leg"), and kick that foot out. Repeat these steps, alternating between the left and right side. *Note: while you are continuously moving forward, you want to have little hops as you alternate sides, so it will not be mere walking.*

Do 20 repetitions, (10 left, 10 right).

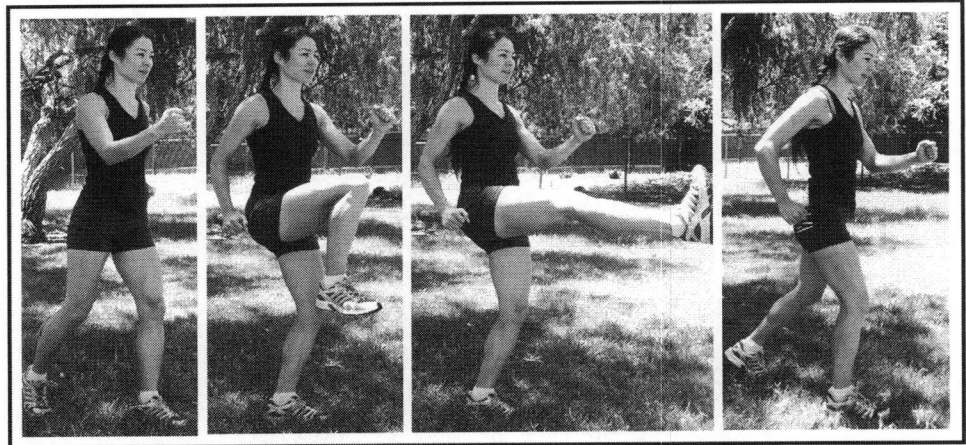

....

Dumbbell Jabs:

Stand with your legs shoulder with apart, in "good standing posture", and remember to keep your knees relaxed. Lift both of your fists to chin level. With controlled movements, alternate punching straight ahead, (lifting the dumbbell to eye level height as you punch), and back to chin level as you retract. Start with 5 lbs, and work your way up to 8lbs.

Do 20 punches total, (10 left, 10 right).

(See photos on the next page)

Dumbbell Jabs

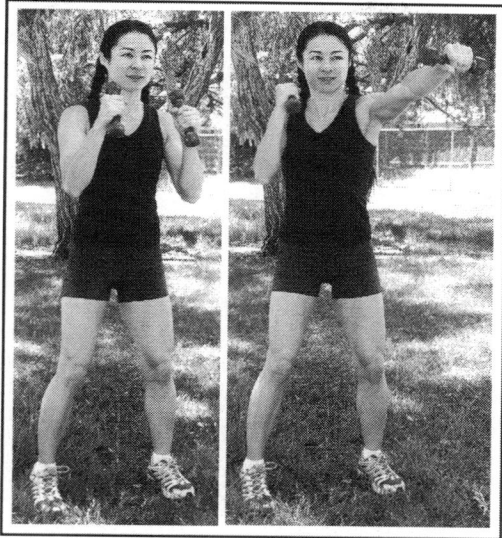

....

Double Leg Hops:

Place both feet close together, (although not touching), and keep your feet like this for the entire exercise. To keep the instructions simple: what you simply do is, consecutive hops forward with both legs. ***Important:*** *As you hop, make sure you keep your knees from buckling, (hitting each other); it is not good for your knees, hips, and ankles.* As you hop, allow your bent elbows to pump forwards and backwards.

Do 20 consecutive hops.

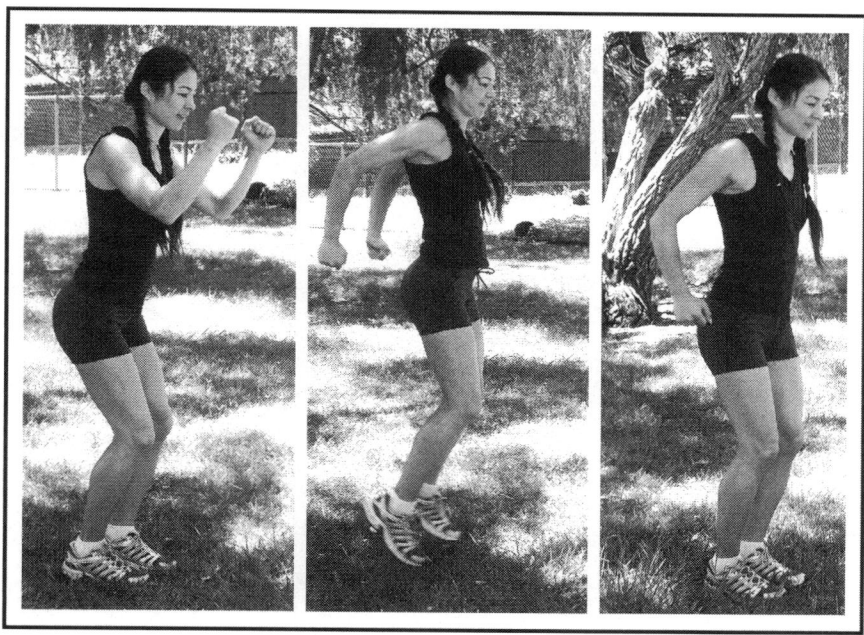

Biceps Curl with Lift:

This is almost exactly like the "Bicep Curls" that you did in Starter Program Level 1; there is just one extra movement at the end.

Stand shoulder width apart, with "good posture". Place your elbows firmly down to your sides. Lift the weights up, and when they are in the "up position", extend your elbows out and up higher, (until the weights are at eye level). Hold for a fraction of a second, then lower your elbows, and then bring your weights back down to the starting position.

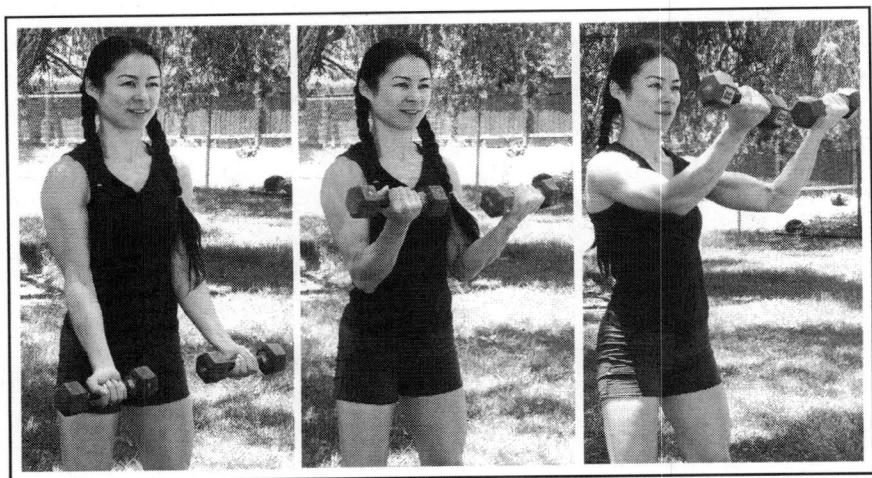

Reminder: as with the regular bicep curls, keep your arms "tight" during the entire set, so you are not resting in the middle of the set.

Important Note: as you lift your weights out and up higher, make sure to breathe out and tighten your abs during this phase. Not only will it help tone your abdominal muscles, it will also make sure you are using your core muscles, as opposed to weight being distributed to you lower back.

Do 8 – 12 repetitions.

Dumbbell Back and Lift:

Hold your dumbbells together, in front of you, slightly above shoulder height level.

Important: make sure you are not hunching your shoulders towards your ears, and have them drawn back and down; this way you are making sure to isolate your shoulder muscles, (which is the intention of this exercise), and you are also strengthening your "good posture" muscles.

Now open up your arms until your dumbbells are slightly behind your back, allowing you chest to open up; you will have a "T" figure. *Reminder: keep your shoulders from "hunching".*

While keeping your arms mostly straight, lift the weights until they lightly touch over your head. *Reminder: again, I can't stress enough on keeping your shoulders back and down the entire time.*

Next, move the dumbbells back down to the "T" figure that you had, then move the dumbbells back to the original start position.

Do 5 repetitions. Use 3 – 5lbs dumbbells.

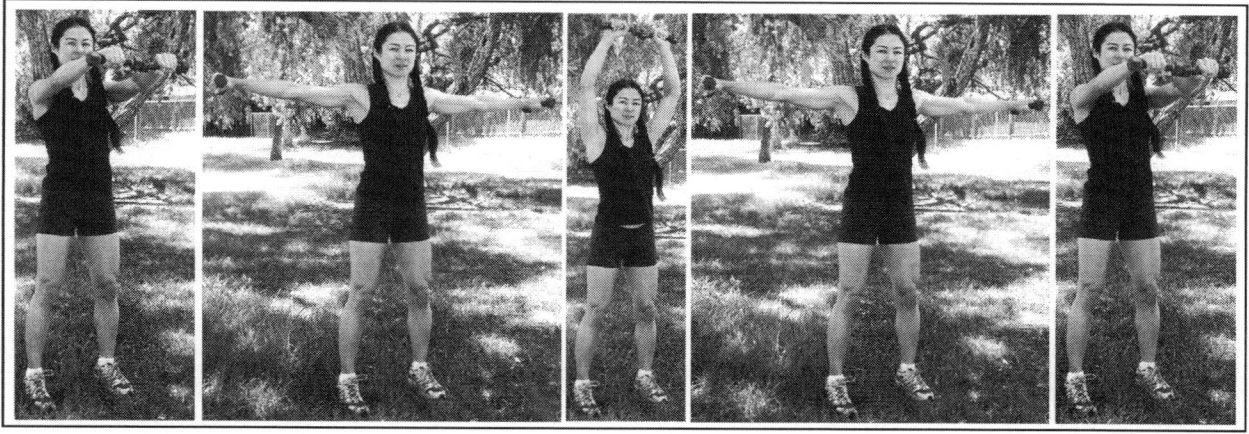

Slides with Twists:

This one will be a tricky one, but once you get it, you will think to yourself, "I can't believe this used to be hard". Be patient, and once you get it, know that you have improved your coordination.

Note: Lets first concentrate on the lower half of your body to begin with, and once you have that down easily, then lets work on your upper body.

You will be continuously moving sideways as you do this exercise, so choose which direction you will be going. **Note:** The leg that's going to be doing most of the "coordination work" will be your "back leg". Your "back leg" is the one that's in the "back" to the direction you will be moving.

Start with your arms and legs open. *Don't think to hard about the upper body because all you will do is make this exercise harder "to get".*

With you "back leg", step behind your "front leg". Then take the "front leg", and open it up so it is leading the way again. This time instead of taking your "back leg" and stepping behind the "front leg", you will step in front of the "front leg". Then as with before, get the "front leg", and open it up so it is leading the way again.

You will continue moving in one direction with the "back leg" alternating with going in front, or behind the "front leg". *(see photos on the next page)*

Do this 15 times in one direction, and without turning around, go back the same direction, (so you can get the other side of your body).

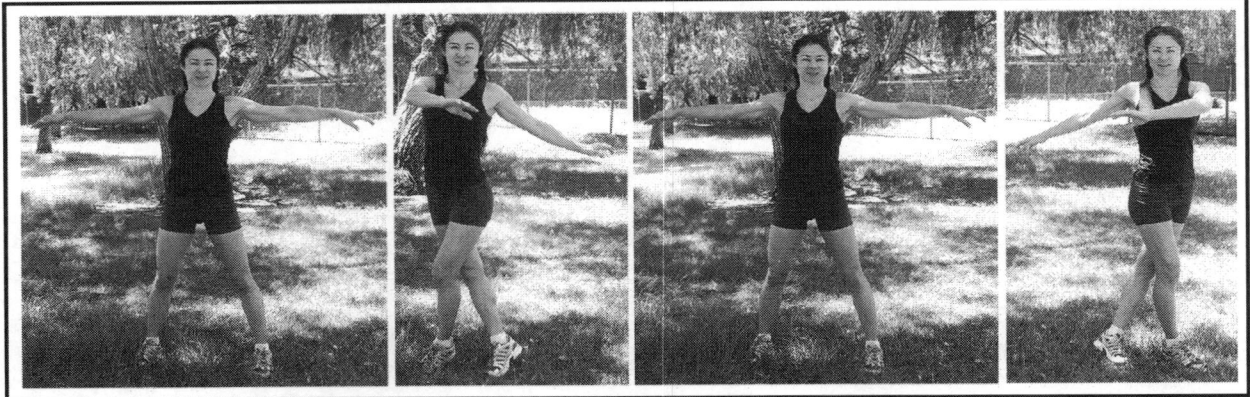

....

<u>Triceps Over-head Press</u>:

Hold tightly with both hands, onto one end of your dumbbell, and spin it around and over your head. Check for "good posture" with your core and shoulders. Keeping your elbows/upper arms fixed in this start position at all times, lift the dumbbell up, then back down. When extending your arms, lift them as straight as possible <u>while</u> squeezing your arms together at the height of extension.

Note: *While your arms are in the bent "start" position, don't relax your arms, so they are not resting in the middle of the set.*

Do 10 repetitions.

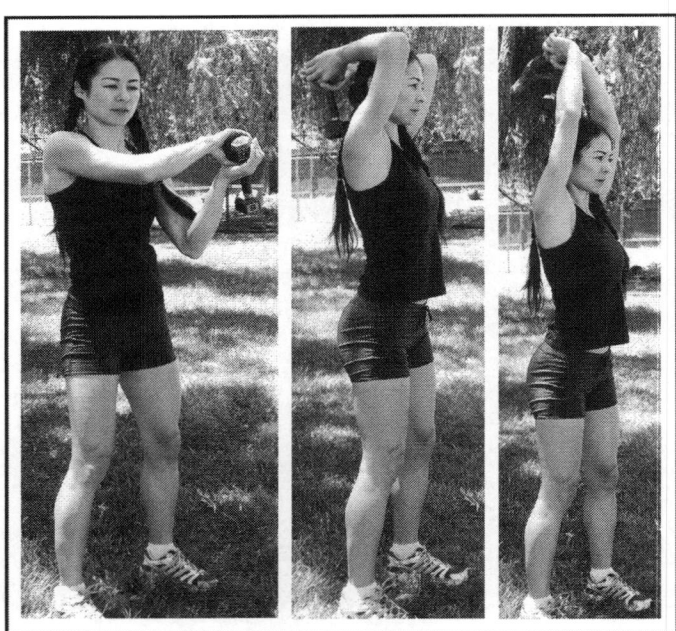

"Full-throttle" Program (level 2)
(running intervals for additional 2 days of training)

* These can be done at a park, or around the neighborhood, and with a baby jogger, or a training partner *

Warm-up:
easy jog - 10 minutes

Intervals:
Sprints On & Offs - 10 sets

Directions:
1. Use a stopwatch.
2. Run at 80 - 90% effort for 1 minute. *Note: It is 80-90% effort, keeping in mind that its for an entire minute, AND keeping in mind that you have 10 of these 1 minutes to do.*
3. After the 1 minute is done, STOP and rest for 1 minute.
Note: Do not sit down, it will make getting up harder, as well, it may cause you to cramp up.
4. Repeat steps #2 and #3 until your have done 10 times, 1 minute sprints.

Cool-down:
easy jog - 5 minutes.

Stretches: standard stretches as noted.

****

Starter Program Level #3:

Standard warm-up: for reminder, refer back to earlier in this chapter.

Circuit:
Jumps squats with Pop outs
Full or Mini Pushups (not on knees)
Front Kicks
Dumbbell Running
Single leg Hops
Isolated Biceps Curls
Dumbbell Pull-ups
Pop Twists
Chair Dips

Standard stretches: for reminder, refer back to earlier in this chapter.

Ishio Method Pelvic Floor Rehab Protocol ᴛᴍ: refer to Ch3 and Ch12, (for the check-off sheets).
Ishio Method Abdominal Rehab Protocol ᴛᴍ: refer to Ch4 and Ch12, (for the check-off sheets).

Jumps Squats with Pop Outs:

These will be a more difficult version of the "Jump Squats" that you did in Starter Program Level 2.

Stand with feet farther than shoulder width apart. As with the jump squats, the first movement you will concentrate on is to move your butt out backwards AS you are bending your knees.

Instead of just touching the ground, and starting back up for another jump, you will "pop" out your feet so you end up in a push-up position.

Options: You can either "walk your legs out", (as in lead with one leg, then the other leg, until both are out in a push-up position), or you can "pop" both of your legs out at the same time.

Once you are in the push-up position, (end position), you want to immediately "pop" your legs back in, (or "walk your legs back in"), then go back to doing a "Jump Squat" as with Level 2.

Start with 3 consecutive Jump Squats with Pops Outs in a row, then a short break, for another set of 3. Your goal is to do 10 consecutive Jump Squats with Pop Outs in a row.

Below is the "walking out" version.

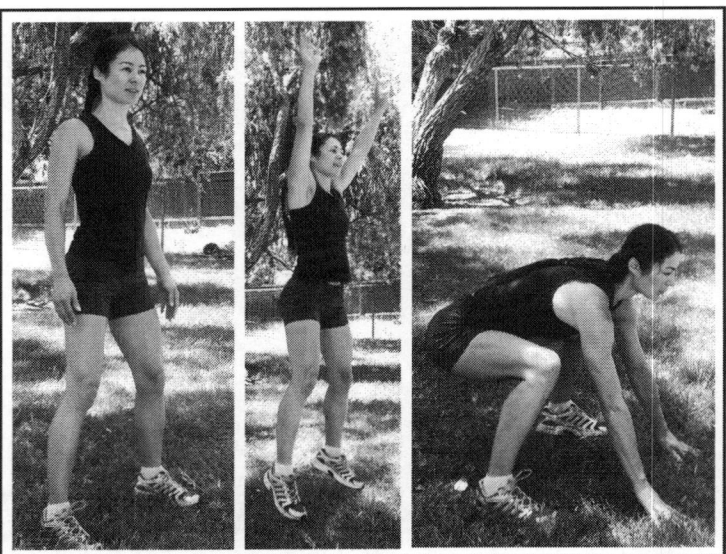
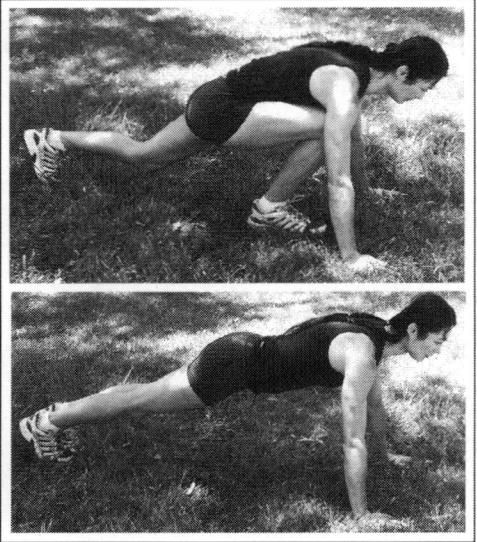

Full or Mini Pushups (basically pushups that are not assisted by being on your knees):

If you haven't done pushups off your knees in the past, it doesn't matter; you will be strong enough to do them off of your knees now.

Important Reminder: shoulders back and down, (not shrugging), chest "opened", wrists directly below your shoulders, keep your abs pulled-in at all times, and your hips from drooping.

With controlled movements, and leading with your chest/torso, bend your arms until you are at a 90degree angle at the elbow. <u>Concentrate on your torso going down</u>, (not so much your mid-section), or you may end up leading with your hips. When leading with your chest, your lower body will automatically follow appropriately, as long as you are keeping your abs and hips taunt in it's position. **If you can't go all the way down to 90 degrees, then do "Mini Pushups".**

Mini Pushups: if you can't go all the way down to 90 degrees at the elbow, then simply don't at this time; go partial way down, and you are now doing "mini pushups". With mini push-ups, you will still be building strength, and as you get stronger, you will be able to go down lower. You will be amazed at how quickly you can start doing full pushups.

Start with 3 reps of Full or Mini Pushups, with a short break, then another set of 3. Build your way up one at a time until you can do 10 in a row.

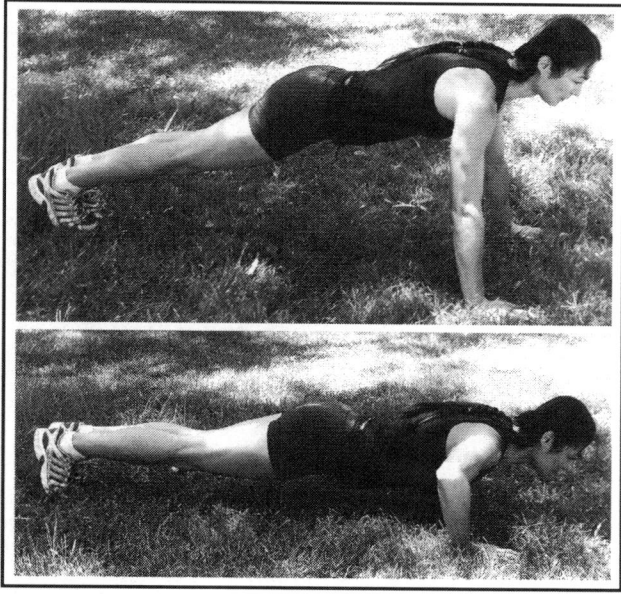

....

Front Kicks:

Start this exercise by kicking to mid-section level, and after you gain strength and flexibility, eventually start kicking higher, until you are kicking at shoulder/head height.

Stand in a "fight stance", like you see in the photo on the next page, (one leg in front of the other, have your feet shoulder width apart). You will be kicking off your back leg for this exercise. Have your back heel slightly lifted off the ground. <u>The first movement you concentrate on when kicking is with lifting your knee up</u>, (not of your foot lifting). Once your knee is lifted, then kick your foot out in front of you. Once you reach full extension with that foot, immediately "recoil" your leg back <u>to the position with your knee bent</u>, BEFORE bringing you leg completely down and back to your starting "fight stance".

Important: Make sure you learn the movements with control before you start going for speed; if not, you can hyper extend your knee, or strain muscles.

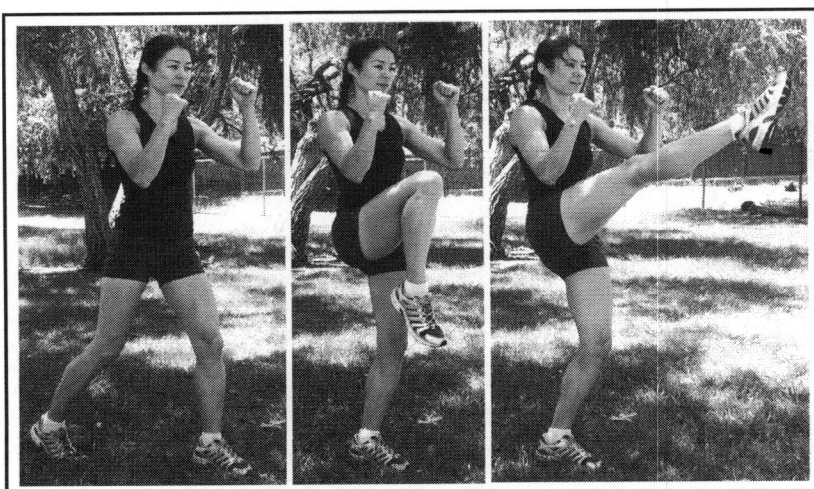

....

<u>Dumbbell Running:</u>

This exercise is especially good for if you are doing the running intervals. Start this exercise at a slower speed, and until you develop great coordination/control with the movements, don't speed up the movements. The goal for this exercise is to increase your speed while maintaining control, not to simply go higher in weight.

Stand with your feet about hip width apart. Slightly bend your knees. Put most of your weight towards the front half of your feet, (so there will be very little to no weight on your heels). Keep your chin slightly down. Start with one arm in front and one behind you, (in a running position). Make sure to keep your elbows at about a 90-degree angle at your elbows at all times. Now move your elbows as if you are running.

Concentrate on moving your elbows back and forth; not the hands. Have good range of motion, bringing your front dumbbell to shoulder height, and the back elbow up as high as comfortably possible in the back.

Do 15 left, 15 right reps for 30 total. Use 3 or 5 lbs. dumbbells.

(see photos on the next page)

Dumbbell Running

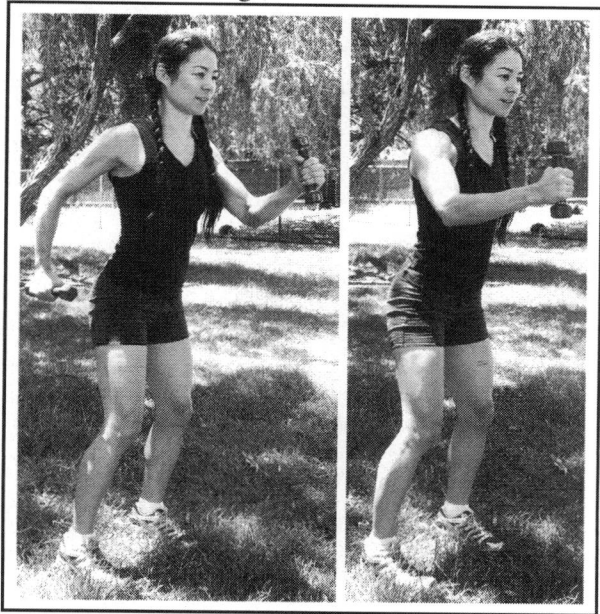

....

Single Leg Hops:

Lift one leg off the ground. To keep the instructions simple: what you simply do is, consecutive hops forward on your single leg.

Important: *As you hop, make sure you keep your knee from buckling, (torqueing inward when you land); it is not good for your knees, hips, and ankles.*

As you hop, allow your arms/elbows to pump forwards and backwards. ***Note:*** *As you build strength and coordination, you can jump higher with each hop.*

Do 10 consecutive hops with one leg, then 10 consecutive hops with the other leg.

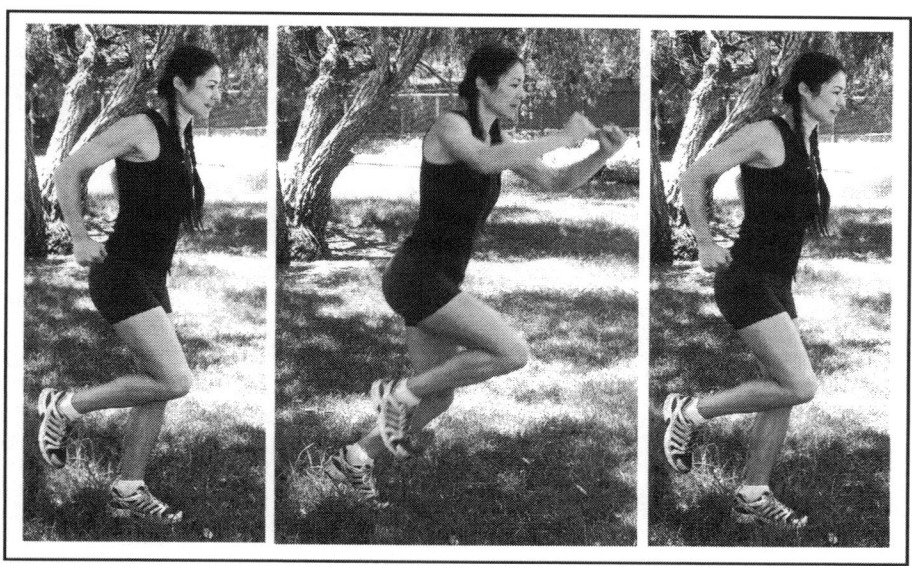

Isolated Biceps Curls:

Sit down on a bench or chair, and scoot forward to the front end of the seat. Lean forward and rest the back of your arm, (the part right above the back of your elbow), against the inside of your thigh, (about a few inches inside from your knee). <u>Without moving your elbow, torso, or shoulder back and forth while lifting</u>, lift your dumbbell up, hold for a fraction of a second, and back down.

Important Note: Don't lift the dumbbell all the way to the very top, (because then your arm will be resting too much), and don't relax your arm when you are at the very bottom of the movement, (because that's also too much resting). <u>Keep your arms tight at all times</u>.

Do 10 reps with the left, 10 reps with the right.

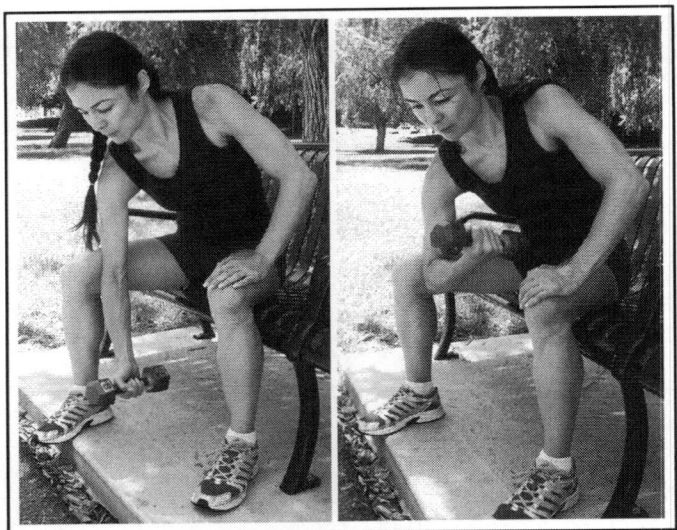

Dumbbell Pull-ups:

Lean forward on a fixed object. Use one arm to hold yourself up (don't lock that arm since you want it to get in some exercise too), and hold the dumbbell in the other hand. With the side that's holding the dumbbell, have that side's leg placed behind you; don't lock that leg either. Keep your back tall, (no hunching).

Now let the arm/shoulder that's holding the dumbbell relax down as far as it will go, (while not slouching over). The <u>first movement it to lift ONLY your shoulder up</u>, and remember not to shrug when doing this, (as with photo number 3 on the next page). After the shoulder is "up", THEN lift your elbow up, bringing the dumbbell next to your hip. Remember to "open" up your chest while lifting your elbow, (so you are really working your upper back). While in control, take your dumbbell back down to the starting position, and repeat.

Do 10 reps on the left, then 10 reps on the right.

Dumbbell Pull-ups   (don't shrug)

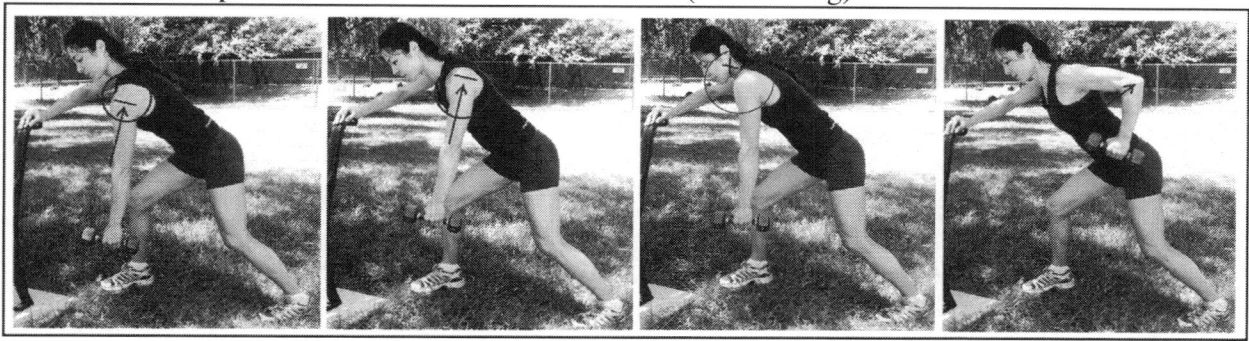

....

Pop Twists:

This is a good workout that helps you become more athletically coordinated, works your core and legs, and gets your heart going. Don't let the directions below intimidate you; it sounds harder to do then if you just try it.

Stand in as comfortable of a wide stance as you can. Now turn your body so it is facing one side, (creating a lead leg feel). Jump up with BOTH legs at the same time, (with the emphasis of your body going UP, not sideways), and while in mid-air, twist your body around so you can land facing the same direction, with your legs having traded sides. Repeat back to the original direction.

Do 10 jumps (alternating between both sides, 5 times each).

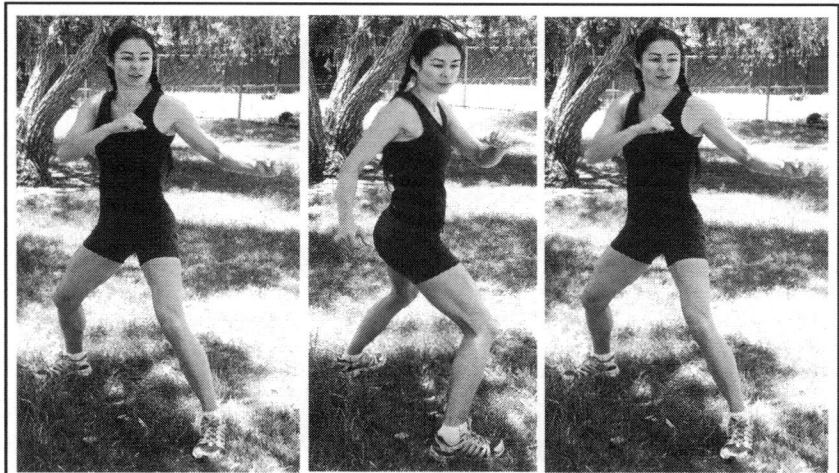

....

Chair Dips:

The straighter you have your legs for this exercise, the more difficult the exercise will be. To start, have your knees bent, and as you become stronger, you can straighten your legs.

While sitting on the bench, place your hands on the bench, (with the top of your fingers facing the same direction as you are sitting). Make sure your hands are placed directly below your shoulders; this will help protect your shoulders. ***Note:*** *depending on your figure, some women will put their hands underneath their hips, while others will simply place their hands next to their hips, (it all depends on your shoulder hip ratio).*

Gently slide off the chair, (bearing your weight on your arms), and adjust your legs to how much you want them to be bent or straight. Now lift your toes so you are on the heels of your feet with the toes going straight up towards the sky. Now <u>draw your shoulders back so your chest is opened</u>. *(see "correct photo" and "incorrect photo" on this and the next page)*

With <u>complete control</u>, bend you elbows so your body is going down; the goal is to have a 90-degree bend at the elbow. ***IMPORTANT:*** *as you bend your elbows, make sure that you keep your elbows going straight back, (as in <u>do not allow your elbows to bow out sideways</u>). Bowing out your elbows can cause pain/problems in the elbows and shoulders.*

Just as **IMPORTANT:** As you go down AND come up, make sure <u>your back stays as close as possible against the bench</u>; this will allow you to properly isolate the triceps and make them do majority of the work as they are supposed to. *Many tend to have their back come way off the bench on the way back up, so be sure to use your legs to help "push" you back towards the bench on the way up.*

Note: if you have your legs straight and are struggling with keeping your elbows from bowing out, and/or your back against the chair, then switch to having your legs bent; as you get stronger, slowly start straightening them back up again.

Another note: if you have your legs bent and are still struggling with form, then don't go all the way down to a 90-degree bend at the elbow, and only go half-way down; once your get stronger, you can start going lower.

Correct: chest opened, and back against bench at all times.

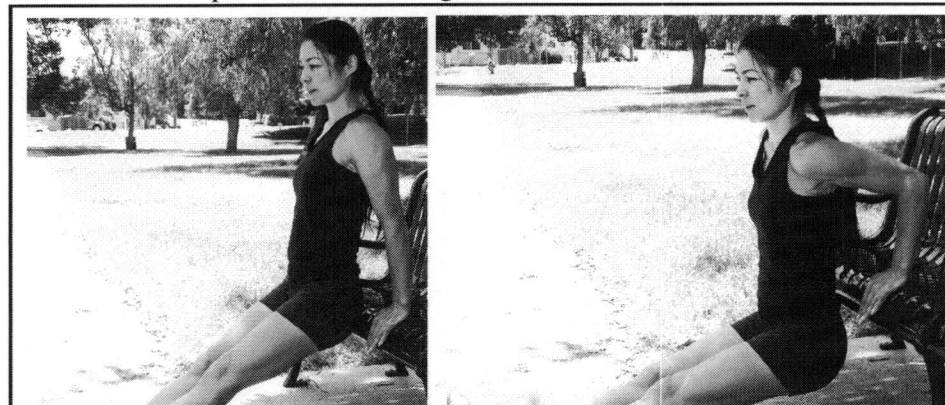

Incorrect: chest collapsed/shoulders hunching, and back is away from bench.

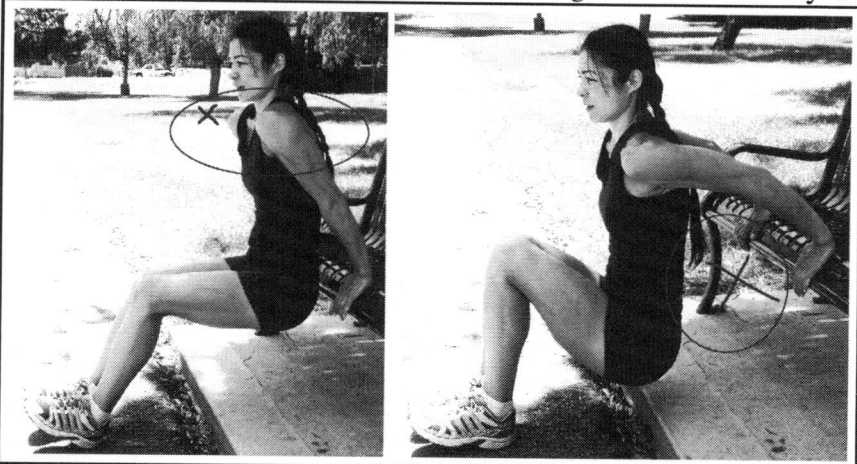

. . . .

"Full-throttle" Program (level 3)
(running intervals for additional 2 days of training)

These can be done at a park/trail with a hill, a hilly block in a neighborhood, or treadmill

Warm-up:
Easy jog- 10 minutes

Intervals:
Hill Repeats - 5 sets

Directions:
1. Use a stopwatch only for the 1ˢᵗ hill rep.

2. Run at 75% effort for 2 minute. *Note: It is 75% effort, keeping in mind that it is continuous running for an entire 2 minutes up hill AND you have 5 of these hills to do.*

3. After running for 2 minutes, STOP. *Remember where you stopped because this will be the same place you stop for the other 4 repetitions.*

4. You recovery is to jog very slowly down the hill, back to your starting point.

5. As soon as you reach the starting point, immediately turn around and do another hill, (with your finish point being where the first repetition's finish point was).

Repeat this hill 5 times.

Cool-down:
Easy jog - 5 minutes.

Stretches: standard stretches as noted.

Golden Rule for Moms

"I AM as IMPORTANT as my children".
Do for ourselves as we do for our children.
It doesn't have to equal the same amount of time,
but it has to equal the same amount of care.

Awareness that you have the ability and responsibility to design the ambiance of your life is powerful wisdom to have; its creativity and productivity are endless.

Chapter Twelve:

Worksheet Tools

Suggestion on how to use work-sheets

For both the Ishio Method – Pelvic Floor Rehab Protocol ™ and Ishio Method – Abdominal Rehab Protocol ™ "Check-off Sheets", use 2 separate **bookmarks** so you can easily locate what week, (page), you are currently on, **or** tear out the pages, and clip them together for easy access.

Tear out the "Lifestyle Log" pages, so you can make copies, and use them month after month.

Tear out the "Workout Check-off" page, so you can make copies, and use them month after month.

Tear out the "Workout Reference", and the "Top-10 Nutrition Favorites" pages, to make copies, so you can make any necessary changes as you progress through your health and fitness needs.

Check-off sheets / Tools

Ishio Method – Pelvic Floor Rehab Exercises Protocol ™ - check-off sheets (pages 178 – 209)

Ishio Method – Abdominal Rehab Exercises Protocol ™ – check-off sheets (pages 210 – 243)

Top 10 Nutrition Favorites Sheet, and example (pages 244 and 245)

Workout Plan Reference Sheet, and example (pages 246 and 247)

Lifestyle Log, and example (pages 248 – 249)

Workout Check-off Sheet (template for copying), and example (pages 253 and 254)

Ishio Method ™ Pelvic Floor Rehab (check-off sheet)

Week 1 (/   /20   thru   /   /20   )

Write in your own personal dates.

Endurance Technique ™

Set: Start - Hold for 10 seconds. Goal - increase in increments of 5 seconds, until sets hold for 20 - 30 seconds.

Day 1 (_____ **)** *write day*

Assessments: *(circle what applies)*
*Surge Posture: 75% or more of the day / 50% of the day / less than 25% of the day
*Core Posture: 75% or more of the day / 50% of the day / less than 25% of the day
Set Posture: 75% or more of the day / 50% of the day / less than 25% of the day
Breathe Posture: 75% or more of the day / 50% of the day / less than 25% of the day

☐ Right after waking up in the morning (3 sets) ☐ Right before bed time. (3 sets)
☐ Every time after using the toilet (1 set each time) ☐ At start of feeding your baby. (1 set each time)
☐ At start of changing baby's diapers. (1 set each time)

Day 2 (_____ **)** *write day*

Assessments: *(circle what applies)*
*Surge Posture: 75% or more of the day / 50% of the day / less than 25% of the day
*Core Posture: 75% or more of the day / 50% of the day / less than 25% of the day
Set Posture: 75% or more of the day / 50% of the day / less than 25% of the day
Breathe Posture: 75% or more of the day / 50% of the day / less than 25% of the day

☐ Right after waking up in the morning (3 sets) ☐ Right before bed time. (3 sets)
☐ Every time after using the toilet (1 set each time) ☐ At start of feeding your baby. (1 set each time)
☐ At start of changing baby's diapers. (1 set each time)

Day 3 (_____ **)** *write day*

Assessments: *(circle what applies)*
*Surge Posture: 75% or more of the day / 50% of the day / less than 25% of the day
*Core Posture: 75% or more of the day / 50% of the day / less than 25% of the day
Set Posture: 75% or more of the day / 50% of the day / less than 25% of the day
Breathe Posture: 75% or more of the day / 50% of the day / less than 25% of the day

☐ Right after waking up in the morning (3 sets) ☐ Right before bed time. (3 sets)
☐ Every time after using the toilet (1 set each time) ☐ At start of feeding your baby. (1 set each time)
☐ At start of changing baby's diapers. (1 set each time)

Day 4 (_____ **)** *write day*

Assessments: *(circle what applies)*
*Surge Posture: 75% or more of the day / 50% of the day / less than 25% of the day
*Core Posture: 75% or more of the day / 50% of the day / less than 25% of the day
Set Posture: 75% or more of the day / 50% of the day / less than 25% of the day
Breathe Posture: 75% or more of the day / 50% of the day / less than 25% of the day

☐ Right after waking up in the morning (3 sets) ☐ Right before bed time. (3 sets)
☐ Every time after using the toilet (1 set each time) ☐ At start of feeding your baby. (1 set each time)
☐ At start of changing baby's diapers. (1 set each time)

Ishio Method ™ Pelvic Floor Rehab (check-off sheet)

Week 1 (/   /20   thru   /   /20   )

Write in your own personal dates.

Endurance Technique ™

Set: Start - Hold for 10 seconds. Goal - increase in increments of 5 seconds, until sets hold for 20 - 30 seconds.

Day 5 (_____ **)** *write day*

Assessments: *(circle what applies)*
*Surge Posture: 75% or more of the day / 50% of the day / less than 25% of the day
*Core Posture: 75% or more of the day / 50% of the day / less than 25% of the day
Set Posture: 75% or more of the day / 50% of the day / less than 25% of the day
Breathe Posture: 75% or more of the day / 50% of the day / less than 25% of the day

☐ Right after waking up in the morning (3 sets)   ☐ Right before bed time. (3 sets)
☐ Every time after using the toilet (1 set each time)   ☐ At start of feeding your baby. (1 set each time)
☐ At start of changing baby's diapers. (1 set each time)

Day 6 (_____ **)** *write day*

Assessments: *(circle what applies)*
*Surge Posture: 75% or more of the day / 50% of the day / less than 25% of the day
*Core Posture: 75% or more of the day / 50% of the day / less than 25% of the day
Set Posture: 75% or more of the day / 50% of the day / less than 25% of the day
Breathe Posture: 75% or more of the day / 50% of the day / less than 25% of the day

☐ Right after waking up in the morning (3 sets)   ☐ Right before bed time. (3 sets)
☐ Every time after using the toilet (1 set each time)   ☐ At start of feeding your baby. (1 set each time)
☐ At start of changing baby's diapers. (1 set each time)

Day 7 (_____ **)** *write day*

Assessments: *(circle what applies)*
*Surge Posture: 75% or more of the day / 50% of the day / less than 25% of the day
*Core Posture: 75% or more of the day / 50% of the day / less than 25% of the day
Set Posture: 75% or more of the day / 50% of the day / less than 25% of the day
Breathe Posture: 75% or more of the day / 50% of the day / less than 25% of the day

☐ Right after waking up in the morning (3 sets)   ☐ Right before bed time. (3 sets)
☐ Every time after using the toilet (1 set each time)   ☐ At start of feeding your baby. (1 set each time)
☐ At start of changing baby's diapers. (1 set each time)

Ishio Method ™ Pelvic Floor Rehab (check-off sheet)

Week 2 (__ / __ /20 thru __ / __ /20)

Write in your own personal dates.

Endurance Technique ™

Set: Start - Hold for 10 seconds. Goal - increase in increments of 5 seconds, until sets hold for 20 - 30 seconds.

Day 1 (_____ **)** *write day*

Assessments: *(circle what applies)*
*Surge Posture: 75% or more of the day / 50% of the day / less than 25% of the day
*Core Posture: 75% or more of the day / 50% of the day / less than 25% of the day
Set Posture: 75% or more of the day / 50% of the day / less than 25% of the day
Breathe Posture: 75% or more of the day / 50% of the day / less than 25% of the day

☐ Right after waking up in the morning (3 sets)   ☐ Right before bed time. (3 sets)
☐ Every time after using the toilet (1 set each time)   ☐ At start of feeding your baby. (1 set each time)
☐ At start of changing baby's diapers. (1 set each time)

Day 2 (_____ **)** *write day*

Assessments: *(circle what applies)*
*Surge Posture: 75% or more of the day / 50% of the day / less than 25% of the day
*Core Posture: 75% or more of the day / 50% of the day / less than 25% of the day
Set Posture: 75% or more of the day / 50% of the day / less than 25% of the day
Breathe Posture: 75% or more of the day / 50% of the day / less than 25% of the day

☐ Right after waking up in the morning (3 sets)   ☐ Right before bed time. (3 sets)
☐ Every time after using the toilet (1 set each time)   ☐ At start of feeding your baby. (1 set each time)
☐ At start of changing baby's diapers. (1 set each time)

Day 3 (_____ **)** *write day*

Assessments: *(circle what applies)*
*Surge Posture: 75% or more of the day / 50% of the day / less than 25% of the day
*Core Posture: 75% or more of the day / 50% of the day / less than 25% of the day
Set Posture: 75% or more of the day / 50% of the day / less than 25% of the day
Breathe Posture: 75% or more of the day / 50% of the day / less than 25% of the day

☐ Right after waking up in the morning (3 sets)   ☐ Right before bed time. (3 sets)
☐ Every time after using the toilet (1 set each time)   ☐ At start of feeding your baby. (1 set each time)
☐ At start of changing baby's diapers. (1 set each time)

Day 4 (_____ **)** *write day*

Assessments: *(circle what applies)*
*Surge Posture: 75% or more of the day / 50% of the day / less than 25% of the day
*Core Posture: 75% or more of the day / 50% of the day / less than 25% of the day
Set Posture: 75% or more of the day / 50% of the day / less than 25% of the day
Breathe Posture: 75% or more of the day / 50% of the day / less than 25% of the day

☐ Right after waking up in the morning (3 sets)   ☐ Right before bed time. (3 sets)
☐ Every time after using the toilet (1 set each time)   ☐ At start of feeding your baby. (1 set each time)
☐ At start of changing baby's diapers. (1 set each time)

Ishio Method ™ Pelvic Floor Rehab (check-off sheet)

Week 2 (/   /20   thru   /   /20   )

Write in your own personal dates.

Endurance Technique ™

Set: Start - Hold for 10 seconds. Goal - increase in increments of 5 seconds, until sets hold for 20 - 30 seconds.

Day 5 (   ) *write day*

Assessments: *(circle what applies)*
*Surge Posture: 75% or more of the day / 50% of the day / less than 25% of the day
*Core Posture: 75% or more of the day / 50% of the day / less than 25% of the day
Set Posture: 75% or more of the day / 50% of the day / less than 25% of the day
Breathe Posture: 75% or more of the day / 50% of the day / less than 25% of the day

☐ Right after waking up in the morning (3 sets)   ☐ Right before bed time. (3 sets)
☐ Every time after using the toilet (1 set each time)   ☐ At start of feeding your baby. (1 set each time)
☐ At start of changing baby's diapers. (1 set each time)

Day 6 (   ) *write day*

Assessments: *(circle what applies)*
*Surge Posture: 75% or more of the day / 50% of the day / less than 25% of the day
*Core Posture: 75% or more of the day / 50% of the day / less than 25% of the day
Set Posture: 75% or more of the day / 50% of the day / less than 25% of the day
Breathe Posture: 75% or more of the day / 50% of the day / less than 25% of the day

☐ Right after waking up in the morning (3 sets)   ☐ Right before bed time. (3 sets)
☐ Every time after using the toilet (1 set each time)   ☐ At start of feeding your baby. (1 set each time)
☐ At start of changing baby's diapers. (1 set each time)

Day 7 (   ) *write day*

Assessments: *(circle what applies)*
*Surge Posture: 75% or more of the day / 50% of the day / less than 25% of the day
*Core Posture: 75% or more of the day / 50% of the day / less than 25% of the day
Set Posture: 75% or more of the day / 50% of the day / less than 25% of the day
Breathe Posture: 75% or more of the day / 50% of the day / less than 25% of the day

☐ Right after waking up in the morning (3 sets)   ☐ Right before bed time. (3 sets)
☐ Every time after using the toilet (1 set each time)   ☐ At start of feeding your baby. (1 set each time)
☐ At start of changing baby's diapers. (1 set each time)

181

Ishio Method ™ Pelvic Floor Rehab (check-off sheet)

Week 3 (/   /20   thru   /   /20   )

Write in your own personal dates.

Endurance Technique ™

Set: Start - Hold for 10 seconds. Goal - increase in increments of 5 seconds, until sets hold for 20 - 30 seconds.

Day 1 (**)** *write day*

Assessments: *(circle what applies)*
*Surge Posture: 75% or more of the day / 50% of the day / less than 25% of the day
*Core Posture: 75% or more of the day / 50% of the day / less than 25% of the day
Set Posture: 75% or more of the day / 50% of the day / less than 25% of the day
Breathe Posture: 75% or more of the day / 50% of the day / less than 25% of the day

☐ Right after waking up in the morning (3 sets)   ☐ Right before bed time. (3 sets)
☐ Every time after using the toilet (1 set each time)   ☐ At start of feeding your baby. (1 set each time)
☐ At start of changing baby's diapers. (1 set each time)

Day 2 (**)** *write day*

Assessments: *(circle what applies)*
*Surge Posture: 75% or more of the day / 50% of the day / less than 25% of the day
*Core Posture: 75% or more of the day / 50% of the day / less than 25% of the day
Set Posture: 75% or more of the day / 50% of the day / less than 25% of the day
Breathe Posture: 75% or more of the day / 50% of the day / less than 25% of the day

☐ Right after waking up in the morning (3 sets)   ☐ Right before bed time. (3 sets)
☐ Every time after using the toilet (1 set each time)   ☐ At start of feeding your baby. (1 set each time)
☐ At start of changing baby's diapers. (1 set each time)

Day 3 (**)** *write day*

Assessments: *(circle what applies)*
*Surge Posture: 75% or more of the day / 50% of the day / less than 25% of the day
*Core Posture: 75% or more of the day / 50% of the day / less than 25% of the day
Set Posture: 75% or more of the day / 50% of the day / less than 25% of the day
Breathe Posture: 75% or more of the day / 50% of the day / less than 25% of the day

☐ Right after waking up in the morning (3 sets)   ☐ Right before bed time. (3 sets)
☐ Every time after using the toilet (1 set each time)   ☐ At start of feeding your baby. (1 set each time)
☐ At start of changing baby's diapers. (1 set each time)

Day 4 (**)** *write day*

Assessments: *(circle what applies)*
*Surge Posture: 75% or more of the day / 50% of the day / less than 25% of the day
*Core Posture: 75% or more of the day / 50% of the day / less than 25% of the day
Set Posture: 75% or more of the day / 50% of the day / less than 25% of the day
Breathe Posture: 75% or more of the day / 50% of the day / less than 25% of the day

☐ Right after waking up in the morning (3 sets)   ☐ Right before bed time. (3 sets)
☐ Every time after using the toilet (1 set each time)   ☐ At start of feeding your baby. (1 set each time)
☐ At start of changing baby's diapers. (1 set each time)

Ishio Method ™ Pelvic Floor Rehab (check-off sheet)

Week 3 (/   /20   thru   /   /20   ) *Write in your own personal dates.*

Endurance Technique ™

Set: Start - Hold for 10 seconds. Goal - increase in increments of 5 seconds, until sets hold for 20 - 30 seconds.

Day 5 (_____ **)** *write day*

Assessments: *(circle what applies)*
*Surge Posture: 75% or more of the day / 50% of the day / less than 25% of the day
*Core Posture: 75% or more of the day / 50% of the day / less than 25% of the day
Set Posture: 75% or more of the day / 50% of the day / less than 25% of the day
Breathe Posture: 75% or more of the day / 50% of the day / less than 25% of the day

☐ Right after waking up in the morning (3 sets)   ☐ Right before bed time. (3 sets)
☐ Every time after using the toilet (1 set each time)   ☐ At start of feeding your baby. (1 set each time)
☐ At start of changing baby's diapers. (1 set each time)

Day 6 (_____ **)** *write day*

Assessments: *(circle what applies)*
*Surge Posture: 75% or more of the day / 50% of the day / less than 25% of the day
*Core Posture: 75% or more of the day / 50% of the day / less than 25% of the day
Set Posture: 75% or more of the day / 50% of the day / less than 25% of the day
Breathe Posture: 75% or more of the day / 50% of the day / less than 25% of the day

☐ Right after waking up in the morning (3 sets)   ☐ Right before bed time. (3 sets)
☐ Every time after using the toilet (1 set each time)   ☐ At start of feeding your baby. (1 set each time)
☐ At start of changing baby's diapers. (1 set each time)

Day 7 (_____ **)** *write day*

Assessments: *(circle what applies)*
*Surge Posture: 75% or more of the day / 50% of the day / less than 25% of the day
*Core Posture: 75% or more of the day / 50% of the day / less than 25% of the day
Set Posture: 75% or more of the day / 50% of the day / less than 25% of the day
Breathe Posture: 75% or more of the day / 50% of the day / less than 25% of the day

☐ Right after waking up in the morning (3 sets)   ☐ Right before bed time. (3 sets)
☐ Every time after using the toilet (1 set each time)   ☐ At start of feeding your baby. (1 set each time)
☐ At start of changing baby's diapers. (1 set each time)

Ishio Method ™ Pelvic Floor Rehab (check-off sheet)

Week 4 (/ /20 thru / /20)

Write in your own personal dates.

Adding: Pulse Technique ™

Set: 10ct / Pull-in 100% and hold (2 sec.), then release slowly without relaxing past 50% of full relaxation, repeat.

Day 1 ( ) *write day*

Assessments: *(circle what applies)*
*Surge Posture: 75% or more of the day / 50% of the day / less than 25% of the day
*Core Posture: 75% or more of the day / 50% of the day / less than 25% of the day
Set Posture: 75% or more of the day / 50% of the day / less than 25% of the day
Breathe Posture: 75% or more of the day / 50% of the day / less than 25% of the day

☐ MORNING: Endurance Technique ™ (1 set), Pulse Technique ™, (2 sets)
☐ AFTERNOON: Endurance Technique ™, (after toilet, start of feeding baby, start of changing baby)
☐ BEFORE BED: Endurance Technnique ™ (1 set), Pulse Technique ™, (2 sets)

Day 2 ( ) *write day*

Assessments: *(circle what applies)*
*Surge Posture: 75% or more of the day / 50% of the day / less than 25% of the day
*Core Posture: 75% or more of the day / 50% of the day / less than 25% of the day
Set Posture: 75% or more of the day / 50% of the day / less than 25% of the day
Breathe Posture: 75% or more of the day / 50% of the day / less than 25% of the day

☐ MORNING: Endurance Technique ™ (1 set), Pulse Technique ™, (2 sets)
☐ AFTERNOON: Endurance Technique ™, (after toilet, start of feeding baby, start of changing baby)
☐ BEFORE BED: Endurance Technnique ™ (1 set), Pulse Technique ™, (2 sets)

Day 3 ( ) *write day*

Assessments: *(circle what applies)*
*Surge Posture: 75% or more of the day / 50% of the day / less than 25% of the day
*Core Posture: 75% or more of the day / 50% of the day / less than 25% of the day
Set Posture: 75% or more of the day / 50% of the day / less than 25% of the day
Breathe Posture: 75% or more of the day / 50% of the day / less than 25% of the day

☐ MORNING: Endurance Technique ™ (1 set), Pulse Technique ™, (2 sets)
☐ AFTERNOON: Endurance Technique ™, (after toilet, start of feeding baby, start of changing baby)
☐ BEFORE BED: Endurance Technnique ™ (1 set), Pulse Technique ™, (2 sets)

Day 4 ( ) *write day*

Assessments: *(circle what applies)*
*Surge Posture: 75% or more of the day / 50% of the day / less than 25% of the day
*Core Posture: 75% or more of the day / 50% of the day / less than 25% of the day
Set Posture: 75% or more of the day / 50% of the day / less than 25% of the day
Breathe Posture: 75% or more of the day / 50% of the day / less than 25% of the day

☐ MORNING: Endurance Technique ™ (1 set), Pulse Technique ™, (2 sets)
☐ AFTERNOON: Endurance Technique ™, (after toilet, start of feeding baby, start of changing baby)
☐ BEFORE BED: Endurance Technnique ™ (1 set), Pulse Technique ™, (2 sets)

Ishio Method ™ Pelvic Floor Rehab (check-off sheet)

Week 4 (/   /20   thru   /   /20   )   *Write in your own personal dates.*

Adding: **Pulse Technique** ™

Set: 10ct / Pull-in 100% and hold (2 sec.), then release slowly without relaxing past 50% of full relaxation, repeat.

Day 5 ( ) *write day*

Assessments: *(circle what applies)*
*Surge Posture: 75% or more of the day / 50% of the day / less than 25% of the day
*Core Posture: 75% or more of the day / 50% of the day / less than 25% of the day
Set Posture: 75% or more of the day / 50% of the day / less than 25% of the day
Breathe Posture: 75% or more of the day / 50% of the day / less than 25% of the day

☐ MORNING: Endurance Technique ™ (1 set), Pulse Technique ™, (2 sets)
☐ AFTERNOON: Endurance Technique ™, (after toilet, start of feeding baby, start of changing baby)
☐ BEFORE BED: Endurance Technnique ™ (1 set), Pulse Technique ™, (2 sets)

Day 6 ( ) *write day*

Assessments: *(circle what applies)*
*Surge Posture: 75% or more of the day / 50% of the day / less than 25% of the day
*Core Posture: 75% or more of the day / 50% of the day / less than 25% of the day
Set Posture: 75% or more of the day / 50% of the day / less than 25% of the day
Breathe Posture: 75% or more of the day / 50% of the day / less than 25% of the day

☐ MORNING: Endurance Technique ™ (1 set), Pulse Technique ™, (2 sets)
☐ AFTERNOON: Endurance Technique ™, (after toilet, start of feeding baby, start of changing baby)
☐ BEFORE BED: Endurance Technnique ™ (1 set), Pulse Technique ™, (2 sets)

Day 7 ( ) *write day*

Assessments: *(circle what applies)*
*Surge Posture: 75% or more of the day / 50% of the day / less than 25% of the day
*Core Posture: 75% or more of the day / 50% of the day / less than 25% of the day
Set Posture: 75% or more of the day / 50% of the day / less than 25% of the day
Breathe Posture: 75% or more of the day / 50% of the day / less than 25% of the day

☐ MORNING: Endurance Technique ™ (1 set), Pulse Technique ™, (2 sets)
☐ AFTERNOON: Endurance Technique ™, (after toilet, start of feeding baby, start of changing baby)
☐ BEFORE BED: Endurance Technnique ™ (1 set), Pulse Technique ™, (2 sets)

Ishio Method ™ Pelvic Floor Rehab (check-off sheet)

Week 5 (/   /20   thru   /   /20   )

Write in your own personal dates.

Adding: **Pulse Technique** ™

Set: 10ct / Pull-in 100% and hold (2 sec.), then release slowly without relaxing past 50% of full relaxation, repeat.

Day 1 (   ) *write day*

Assessments: *(circle what applies)*
*Surge Posture: 75% or more of the day / 50% of the day / less than 25% of the day
*Core Posture: 75% or more of the day / 50% of the day / less than 25% of the day
Set Posture: 75% or more of the day / 50% of the day / less than 25% of the day
Breathe Posture: 75% or more of the day / 50% of the day / less than 25% of the day

☐ MORNING: Endurance Technique ™ (1 set), Pulse Technique ™, (2 sets)
☐ AFTERNOON: Endurance Technique ™, (after toilet, start of feeding baby, start of changing baby)
☐ BEFORE BED: Endurance Technnique ™ (1 set), Pulse Technique ™, (2 sets)

Day 2 (   ) *write day*

Assessments: *(circle what applies)*
*Surge Posture: 75% or more of the day / 50% of the day / less than 25% of the day
*Core Posture: 75% or more of the day / 50% of the day / less than 25% of the day
Set Posture: 75% or more of the day / 50% of the day / less than 25% of the day
Breathe Posture: 75% or more of the day / 50% of the day / less than 25% of the day

☐ MORNING: Endurance Technique ™ (1 set), Pulse Technique ™, (2 sets)
☐ AFTERNOON: Endurance Technique ™, (after toilet, start of feeding baby, start of changing baby)
☐ BEFORE BED: Endurance Technnique ™ (1 set), Pulse Technique ™, (2 sets)

Day 3 (   ) *write day*

Assessments: *(circle what applies)*
*Surge Posture: 75% or more of the day / 50% of the day / less than 25% of the day
*Core Posture: 75% or more of the day / 50% of the day / less than 25% of the day
Set Posture: 75% or more of the day / 50% of the day / less than 25% of the day
Breathe Posture: 75% or more of the day / 50% of the day / less than 25% of the day

☐ MORNING: Endurance Technique ™ (1 set), Pulse Technique ™, (2 sets)
☐ AFTERNOON: Endurance Technique ™, (after toilet, start of feeding baby, start of changing baby)
☐ BEFORE BED: Endurance Technnique ™ (1 set), Pulse Technique ™, (2 sets)

Day 4 (   ) *write day*

Assessments: *(circle what applies)*
*Surge Posture: 75% or more of the day / 50% of the day / less than 25% of the day
*Core Posture: 75% or more of the day / 50% of the day / less than 25% of the day
Set Posture: 75% or more of the day / 50% of the day / less than 25% of the day
Breathe Posture: 75% or more of the day / 50% of the day / less than 25% of the day

☐ MORNING: Endurance Technique ™ (1 set), Pulse Technique ™, (2 sets)
☐ AFTERNOON: Endurance Technique ™, (after toilet, start of feeding baby, start of changing baby)
☐ BEFORE BED: Endurance Technnique ™ (1 set), Pulse Technique ™, (2 sets)

186

Ishio Method ™ Pelvic Floor Rehab (check-off sheet)

Week 5 (/   /20   thru   /   /20   )

Write in your own personal dates.

Adding: **Pulse Technique** ™

Set: 10ct / Pull-in 100% and hold (2 sec.), then release slowly without relaxing past 50% of full relaxation, repeat.

Day 5 (   ) *write day*

Assessments: *(circle what applies)*
*Surge Posture: 75% or more of the day / 50% of the day / less than 25% of the day
*Core Posture: 75% or more of the day / 50% of the day / less than 25% of the day
Set Posture: 75% or more of the day / 50% of the day / less than 25% of the day
Breathe Posture: 75% or more of the day / 50% of the day / less than 25% of the day

☐ MORNING: Endurance Technique ™ (1 set), Pulse Technique ™, (2 sets)
☐ AFTERNOON: Endurance Technique ™, (after toilet, start of feeding baby, start of changing baby)
☐ BEFORE BED: Endurance Technnique ™ (1 set), Pulse Technique ™, (2 sets)

Day 6 (   ) *write day*

Assessments: *(circle what applies)*
*Surge Posture: 75% or more of the day / 50% of the day / less than 25% of the day
*Core Posture: 75% or more of the day / 50% of the day / less than 25% of the day
Set Posture: 75% or more of the day / 50% of the day / less than 25% of the day
Breathe Posture: 75% or more of the day / 50% of the day / less than 25% of the day

☐ MORNING: Endurance Technique ™ (1 set), Pulse Technique ™, (2 sets)
☐ AFTERNOON: Endurance Technique ™, (after toilet, start of feeding baby, start of changing baby)
☐ BEFORE BED: Endurance Technnique ™ (1 set), Pulse Technique ™, (2 sets)

Day 7 (   ) *write day*

Assessments: *(circle what applies)*
*Surge Posture: 75% or more of the day / 50% of the day / less than 25% of the day
*Core Posture: 75% or more of the day / 50% of the day / less than 25% of the day
Set Posture: 75% or more of the day / 50% of the day / less than 25% of the day
Breathe Posture: 75% or more of the day / 50% of the day / less than 25% of the day

☐ MORNING: Endurance Technique ™ (1 set), Pulse Technique ™, (2 sets)
☐ AFTERNOON: Endurance Technique ™, (after toilet, start of feeding baby, start of changing baby)
☐ BEFORE BED: Endurance Technnique ™ (1 set), Pulse Technique ™, (2 sets)

Ishio Method ™ Pelvic Floor Rehab (check-off sheet)

Week 6 (/   /20   thru   /   /20   )   *Write in your own personal dates.*

Adding: **Pulse Technique** ™

Set: 10ct / Pull-in 100% and hold (2 sec.), then release slowly without relaxing past 50% of full relaxation, repeat.

Day 1 (   ) *write day*

Assessments: *(circle what applies)*
*Surge Posture: 75% or more of the day / 50% of the day / less than 25% of the day
*Core Posture: 75% or more of the day / 50% of the day / less than 25% of the day
Set Posture: 75% or more of the day / 50% of the day / less than 25% of the day
Breathe Posture: 75% or more of the day / 50% of the day / less than 25% of the day

☐ MORNING: Endurance Technique ™ (1 set), Pulse Technique ™, (2 sets)
☐ AFTERNOON: Endurance Technique ™, (after toilet, start of feeding baby, start of changing baby)
☐ BEFORE BED: Endurance Technnique ™ (1 set), Pulse Technique ™, (2 sets)

Day 2 (   ) *write day*

Assessments: *(circle what applies)*
*Surge Posture: 75% or more of the day / 50% of the day / less than 25% of the day
*Core Posture: 75% or more of the day / 50% of the day / less than 25% of the day
Set Posture: 75% or more of the day / 50% of the day / less than 25% of the day
Breathe Posture: 75% or more of the day / 50% of the day / less than 25% of the day

☐ MORNING: Endurance Technique ™ (1 set), Pulse Technique ™, (2 sets)
☐ AFTERNOON: Endurance Technique ™, (after toilet, start of feeding baby, start of changing baby)
☐ BEFORE BED: Endurance Technnique ™ (1 set), Pulse Technique ™, (2 sets)

Day 3 (   ) *write day*

Assessments: *(circle what applies)*
*Surge Posture: 75% or more of the day / 50% of the day / less than 25% of the day
*Core Posture: 75% or more of the day / 50% of the day / less than 25% of the day
Set Posture: 75% or more of the day / 50% of the day / less than 25% of the day
Breathe Posture: 75% or more of the day / 50% of the day / less than 25% of the day

☐ MORNING: Endurance Technique ™ (1 set), Pulse Technique ™, (2 sets)
☐ AFTERNOON: Endurance Technique ™, (after toilet, start of feeding baby, start of changing baby)
☐ BEFORE BED: Endurance Technnique ™ (1 set), Pulse Technique ™, (2 sets)

Day 4 (   ) *write day*

Assessments: *(circle what applies)*
*Surge Posture: 75% or more of the day / 50% of the day / less than 25% of the day
*Core Posture: 75% or more of the day / 50% of the day / less than 25% of the day
Set Posture: 75% or more of the day / 50% of the day / less than 25% of the day
Breathe Posture: 75% or more of the day / 50% of the day / less than 25% of the day

☐ MORNING: Endurance Technique ™ (1 set), Pulse Technique ™, (2 sets)
☐ AFTERNOON: Endurance Technique ™, (after toilet, start of feeding baby, start of changing baby)
☐ BEFORE BED: Endurance Technnique ™ (1 set), Pulse Technique ™, (2 sets)

188

Ishio Method ™ Pelvic Floor Rehab (check-off sheet)

Week 6 (/   /20   thru   /   /20   )

Write in your own personal dates.

Adding: **Pulse Technique** ™

Set: 10ct / Pull-in 100% and hold (2 sec.), then release slowly without relaxing past 50% of full relaxation, repeat.

Day 5 (_____ **)** *write day*

Assessments: *(circle what applies)*
*Surge Posture: 75% or more of the day / 50% of the day / less than 25% of the day
*Core Posture: 75% or more of the day / 50% of the day / less than 25% of the day
Set Posture: 75% or more of the day / 50% of the day / less than 25% of the day
Breathe Posture: 75% or more of the day / 50% of the day / less than 25% of the day

☐ MORNING: Endurance Technique ™ (1 set), Pulse Technique ™, (2 sets)
☐ AFTERNOON: Endurance Technique ™, (after toilet, start of feeding baby, start of changing baby)
☐ BEFORE BED: Endurance Technnique ™ (1 set), Pulse Technique ™, (2 sets)

Day 6 (_____ **)** *write day*

Assessments: *(circle what applies)*
*Surge Posture: 75% or more of the day / 50% of the day / less than 25% of the day
*Core Posture: 75% or more of the day / 50% of the day / less than 25% of the day
Set Posture: 75% or more of the day / 50% of the day / less than 25% of the day
Breathe Posture: 75% or more of the day / 50% of the day / less than 25% of the day

☐ MORNING: Endurance Technique ™ (1 set), Pulse Technique ™, (2 sets)
☐ AFTERNOON: Endurance Technique ™, (after toilet, start of feeding baby, start of changing baby)
☐ BEFORE BED: Endurance Technnique ™ (1 set), Pulse Technique ™, (2 sets)

Day 7 (_____ **)** *write day*

Assessments: *(circle what applies)*
*Surge Posture: 75% or more of the day / 50% of the day / less than 25% of the day
*Core Posture: 75% or more of the day / 50% of the day / less than 25% of the day
Set Posture: 75% or more of the day / 50% of the day / less than 25% of the day
Breathe Posture: 75% or more of the day / 50% of the day / less than 25% of the day

☐ MORNING: Endurance Technique ™ (1 set), Pulse Technique ™, (2 sets)
☐ AFTERNOON: Endurance Technique ™, (after toilet, start of feeding baby, start of changing baby)
☐ BEFORE BED: Endurance Technnique ™ (1 set), Pulse Technique ™, (2 sets)

Ishio Method ™ Pelvic Floor Rehab (check-off sheet)

Week 7 (/   /20   thru   /   /20   )   *Write in your own personal dates.*

Adding: **Popins Technique** ™

Set: 10ct / "Pull-in" 100%, (for a fraction of a second), then immediately relax only up to 50%, (for only a fraction of a second), and repeat.

Day 1 ( ) *write day*

Assessments: *(circle what applies)*
*Surge Posture: 75% or more of the day / 50% of the day / less than 25% of the day
*Core Posture: 75% or more of the day / 50% of the day / less than 25% of the day
Set Posture: 75% or more of the day / 50% of the day / less than 25% of the day
Breathe Posture: 75% or more of the day / 50% of the day / less than 25% of the day

☐ MORNING: Endurance Technique ™ (1 set), Pulse Technique ™, (1 set), Popins Technique (2 sets).
☐ AFTERNOON: Endurance Technique ™, (after toilet, start of feeding baby, start of changing baby)
☐ BEFORE BED: Endurance ™ (1 set), Pulse ™, (1 set), Popins ™, (in recommended Anti-Gravity Position ™)

Day 2 ( ) *write day*

Assessments: *(circle what applies)*
*Surge Posture: 75% or more of the day / 50% of the day / less than 25% of the day
*Core Posture: 75% or more of the day / 50% of the day / less than 25% of the day
Set Posture: 75% or more of the day / 50% of the day / less than 25% of the day
Breathe Posture: 75% or more of the day / 50% of the day / less than 25% of the day

☐ MORNING: Endurance Technique ™ (1 set), Pulse Technique ™, (1 set), Popins Technique (2 sets).
☐ AFTERNOON: Endurance Technique ™, (after toilet, start of feeding baby, start of changing baby)
☐ BEFORE BED: Endurance ™ (1 set), Pulse ™, (1 set), Popins ™, (in recommended Anti-Gravity Position ™)

Day 3 ( ) *write day*

Assessments: *(circle what applies)*
*Surge Posture: 75% or more of the day / 50% of the day / less than 25% of the day
*Core Posture: 75% or more of the day / 50% of the day / less than 25% of the day
Set Posture: 75% or more of the day / 50% of the day / less than 25% of the day
Breathe Posture: 75% or more of the day / 50% of the day / less than 25% of the day

☐ MORNING: Endurance Technique ™ (1 set), Pulse Technique ™, (1 set), Popins Technique (2 sets).
☐ AFTERNOON: Endurance Technique ™, (after toilet, start of feeding baby, start of changing baby)
☐ BEFORE BED: Endurance ™ (1 set), Pulse ™, (1 set), Popins ™, (in recommended Anti-Gravity Position ™)

Day 4 ( ) *write day*

Assessments: *(circle what applies)*
*Surge Posture: 75% or more of the day / 50% of the day / less than 25% of the day
*Core Posture: 75% or more of the day / 50% of the day / less than 25% of the day
Set Posture: 75% or more of the day / 50% of the day / less than 25% of the day
Breathe Posture: 75% or more of the day / 50% of the day / less than 25% of the day

☐ MORNING: Endurance Technique ™ (1 set), Pulse Technique ™, (1 set), Popins Technique (2 sets).
☐ AFTERNOON: Endurance Technique ™, (after toilet, start of feeding baby, start of changing baby)
☐ BEFORE BED: Endurance ™ (1 set), Pulse ™, (1 set), Popins ™, (in recommended Anti-Gravity Position ™)

Ishio Method ™ Pelvic Floor Rehab (check-off sheet)

Week 7 (/   /20   thru   /   /20   )

Write in your own personal dates.

Adding: Popins Technique ™

Set: 10ct / "Pull-in" 100%, (for a fraction of a second), then immediately relax only up to 50%, (for only a fraction of a second), and repeat.

Day 5 (   ) *write day*

Assessments: *(circle what applies)*
*Surge Posture: 75% or more of the day / 50% of the day / less than 25% of the day
*Core Posture: 75% or more of the day / 50% of the day / less than 25% of the day
Set Posture: 75% or more of the day / 50% of the day / less than 25% of the day
Breathe Posture: 75% or more of the day / 50% of the day / less than 25% of the day

☐ MORNING: Endurance Technique ™ (1 set), Pulse Technique ™, (1 set), Popins Technique (2 sets).
☐ AFTERNOON: Endurance Technique ™, (after toilet, start of feeding baby, start of changing baby)
☐ BEFORE BED: Endurance ™ (1 set), Pulse ™, (1 set), Popins ™, (in recommended Anti-Gravity Position ™)

Day 6 (   ) *write day*

Assessments: *(circle what applies)*
*Surge Posture: 75% or more of the day / 50% of the day / less than 25% of the day
*Core Posture: 75% or more of the day / 50% of the day / less than 25% of the day
Set Posture: 75% or more of the day / 50% of the day / less than 25% of the day
Breathe Posture: 75% or more of the day / 50% of the day / less than 25% of the day

☐ MORNING: Endurance Technique ™ (1 set), Pulse Technique ™, (1 set), Popins Technique (2 sets).
☐ AFTERNOON: Endurance Technique ™, (after toilet, start of feeding baby, start of changing baby)
☐ BEFORE BED: Endurance ™ (1 set), Pulse ™, (1 set), Popins ™, (in recommended Anti-Gravity Position ™)

Day 7 (   ) *write day*

Assessments: *(circle what applies)*
*Surge Posture: 75% or more of the day / 50% of the day / less than 25% of the day
*Core Posture: 75% or more of the day / 50% of the day / less than 25% of the day
Set Posture: 75% or more of the day / 50% of the day / less than 25% of the day
Breathe Posture: 75% or more of the day / 50% of the day / less than 25% of the day

☐ MORNING: Endurance Technique ™ (1 set), Pulse Technique ™, (1 set), Popins Technique (2 sets).
☐ AFTERNOON: Endurance Technique ™, (after toilet, start of feeding baby, start of changing baby)
☐ BEFORE BED: Endurance ™ (1 set), Pulse ™, (1 set), Popins ™, (in recommended Anti-Gravity Position ™)

Ishio Method ™ Pelvic Floor Rehab (check-off sheet)

Week 8 (/   /20   thru   /   /20   ) *Write in your own personal dates.*

Adding: **Popins Technique** ™

Set: 10ct / "Pull-in" 100%, (for a fraction of a second), then immediately relax only up to 50%, (for only a fraction of a second), and repeat.

Day 1 (**)** *write day*

Assessments: *(circle what applies)*
*Surge Posture: 75% or more of the day / 50% of the day / less than 25% of the day
*Core Posture: 75% or more of the day / 50% of the day / less than 25% of the day
Set Posture: 75% or more of the day / 50% of the day / less than 25% of the day
Breathe Posture: 75% or more of the day / 50% of the day / less than 25% of the day

☐ MORNING: Endurance Technique ™ (1 set), Pulse Technique ™, (1 set), Popins Technique (2 sets).
☐ AFTERNOON: Endurance Technique ™, (after toilet, start of feeding baby, start of changing baby)
☐ BEFORE BED: Endurance ™ (1 set), Pulse ™, (1 set), Popins ™, (in recommended Anti-Gravity Position ™)

Day 2 (**)** *write day*

Assessments: *(circle what applies)*
*Surge Posture: 75% or more of the day / 50% of the day / less than 25% of the day
*Core Posture: 75% or more of the day / 50% of the day / less than 25% of the day
Set Posture: 75% or more of the day / 50% of the day / less than 25% of the day
Breathe Posture: 75% or more of the day / 50% of the day / less than 25% of the day

☐ MORNING: Endurance Technique ™ (1 set), Pulse Technique ™, (1 set), Popins Technique (2 sets).
☐ AFTERNOON: Endurance Technique ™, (after toilet, start of feeding baby, start of changing baby)
☐ BEFORE BED: Endurance ™ (1 set), Pulse ™, (1 set), Popins ™, (in recommended Anti-Gravity Position ™)

Day 3 (**)** *write day*

Assessments: *(circle what applies)*
*Surge Posture: 75% or more of the day / 50% of the day / less than 25% of the day
*Core Posture: 75% or more of the day / 50% of the day / less than 25% of the day
Set Posture: 75% or more of the day / 50% of the day / less than 25% of the day
Breathe Posture: 75% or more of the day / 50% of the day / less than 25% of the day

☐ MORNING: Endurance Technique ™ (1 set), Pulse Technique ™, (1 set), Popins Technique (2 sets).
☐ AFTERNOON: Endurance Technique ™, (after toilet, start of feeding baby, start of changing baby)
☐ BEFORE BED: Endurance ™ (1 set), Pulse ™, (1 set), Popins ™, (in recommended Anti-Gravity Position ™)

Day 4 (**)** *write day*

Assessments: *(circle what applies)*
*Surge Posture: 75% or more of the day / 50% of the day / less than 25% of the day
*Core Posture: 75% or more of the day / 50% of the day / less than 25% of the day
Set Posture: 75% or more of the day / 50% of the day / less than 25% of the day
Breathe Posture: 75% or more of the day / 50% of the day / less than 25% of the day

☐ MORNING: Endurance Technique ™ (1 set), Pulse Technique ™, (1 set), Popins Technique (2 sets).
☐ AFTERNOON: Endurance Technique ™, (after toilet, start of feeding baby, start of changing baby)
☐ BEFORE BED: Endurance ™ (1 set), Pulse ™, (1 set), Popins ™, (in recommended Anti-Gravity Position ™)

Ishio Method ™ Pelvic Floor Rehab (check-off sheet)

Week 8 (/   /20   thru   /   /20   )

Write in your own personal dates.

Adding: Popins Technique ™

Set: 10ct / "Pull-in" 100%, (for a fraction of a second), then immediately relax only up to 50%, (for only a fraction of a second), and repeat.

Day 5 (_____ **)** *write day*

Assessments: *(circle what applies)*
*Surge Posture: 75% or more of the day / 50% of the day / less than 25% of the day
*Core Posture: 75% or more of the day / 50% of the day / less than 25% of the day
Set Posture: 75% or more of the day / 50% of the day / less than 25% of the day
Breathe Posture: 75% or more of the day / 50% of the day / less than 25% of the day

☐ MORNING: Endurance Technique ™ (1 set), Pulse Technique ™, (1 set), Popins Technique (2 sets).
☐ AFTERNOON: Endurance Technique ™, (after toilet, start of feeding baby, start of changing baby)
☐ BEFORE BED: Endurance ™ (1 set), Pulse ™, (1 set), Popins ™, (in recommended Anti-Gravity Position ™)

Day 6 (_____ **)** *write day*

Assessments: *(circle what applies)*
*Surge Posture: 75% or more of the day / 50% of the day / less than 25% of the day
*Core Posture: 75% or more of the day / 50% of the day / less than 25% of the day
Set Posture: 75% or more of the day / 50% of the day / less than 25% of the day
Breathe Posture: 75% or more of the day / 50% of the day / less than 25% of the day

☐ MORNING: Endurance Technique ™ (1 set), Pulse Technique ™, (1 set), Popins Technique (2 sets).
☐ AFTERNOON: Endurance Technique ™, (after toilet, start of feeding baby, start of changing baby)
☐ BEFORE BED: Endurance ™ (1 set), Pulse ™, (1 set), Popins ™, (in recommended Anti-Gravity Position ™)

Day 7 (_____ **)** *write day*

Assessments: *(circle what applies)*
*Surge Posture: 75% or more of the day / 50% of the day / less than 25% of the day
*Core Posture: 75% or more of the day / 50% of the day / less than 25% of the day
Set Posture: 75% or more of the day / 50% of the day / less than 25% of the day
Breathe Posture: 75% or more of the day / 50% of the day / less than 25% of the day

☐ MORNING: Endurance Technique ™ (1 set), Pulse Technique ™, (1 set), Popins Technique (2 sets).
☐ AFTERNOON: Endurance Technique ™, (after toilet, start of feeding baby, start of changing baby)
☐ BEFORE BED: Endurance ™ (1 set), Pulse ™, (1 set), Popins ™, (in recommended Anti-Gravity Position ™)

Ishio Method ™ Pelvic Floor Rehab (check-off sheet)

Week 9 (/   /20   thru   /   /20   )

Write in your own personal dates.

Adding: **Popins Technique** ™

Set: 10ct / "Pull-in" 100%, (for a fraction of a second), then immediately relax only up to 50%, (for only a fraction of a second), and repeat.

Day 1 (   ) write day

Assessments: *(circle what applies)*
*Surge Posture: 75% or more of the day / 50% of the day / less than 25% of the day
*Core Posture: 75% or more of the day / 50% of the day / less than 25% of the day
Set Posture: 75% or more of the day / 50% of the day / less than 25% of the day
Breathe Posture: 75% or more of the day / 50% of the day / less than 25% of the day

☐ MORNING: Endurance Technique ™ (1 set), Pulse Technique ™, (1 set), Popins Technique (2 sets).
☐ AFTERNOON: Endurance Technique ™, (after toilet, start of feeding baby, start of changing baby)
☐ BEFORE BED: Endurance ™ (1 set), Pulse ™, (1 set), Popins ™, (in recommended Anti-Gravity Position ™)

Day 2 (   ) write day

Assessments: *(circle what applies)*
*Surge Posture: 75% or more of the day / 50% of the day / less than 25% of the day
*Core Posture: 75% or more of the day / 50% of the day / less than 25% of the day
Set Posture: 75% or more of the day / 50% of the day / less than 25% of the day
Breathe Posture: 75% or more of the day / 50% of the day / less than 25% of the day

☐ MORNING: Endurance Technique ™ (1 set), Pulse Technique ™, (1 set), Popins Technique (2 sets).
☐ AFTERNOON: Endurance Technique ™, (after toilet, start of feeding baby, start of changing baby)
☐ BEFORE BED: Endurance ™ (1 set), Pulse ™, (1 set), Popins ™, (in recommended Anti-Gravity Position ™)

Day 3 (   ) write day

Assessments: *(circle what applies)*
*Surge Posture: 75% or more of the day / 50% of the day / less than 25% of the day
*Core Posture: 75% or more of the day / 50% of the day / less than 25% of the day
Set Posture: 75% or more of the day / 50% of the day / less than 25% of the day
Breathe Posture: 75% or more of the day / 50% of the day / less than 25% of the day

☐ MORNING: Endurance Technique ™ (1 set), Pulse Technique ™, (1 set), Popins Technique (2 sets).
☐ AFTERNOON: Endurance Technique ™, (after toilet, start of feeding baby, start of changing baby)
☐ BEFORE BED: Endurance ™ (1 set), Pulse ™, (1 set), Popins ™, (in recommended Anti-Gravity Position ™)

Day 4 (   ) write day

Assessments: *(circle what applies)*
*Surge Posture: 75% or more of the day / 50% of the day / less than 25% of the day
*Core Posture: 75% or more of the day / 50% of the day / less than 25% of the day
Set Posture: 75% or more of the day / 50% of the day / less than 25% of the day
Breathe Posture: 75% or more of the day / 50% of the day / less than 25% of the day

☐ MORNING: Endurance Technique ™ (1 set), Pulse Technique ™, (1 set), Popins Technique (2 sets).
☐ AFTERNOON: Endurance Technique ™, (after toilet, start of feeding baby, start of changing baby)
☐ BEFORE BED: Endurance ™ (1 set), Pulse ™, (1 set), Popins ™, (in recommended Anti-Gravity Position ™)

Ishio Method ™ Pelvic Floor Rehab (check-off sheet)

Week 9 (/   /20   thru   /   /20   )

Write in your own personal dates.

Adding: Popins Technique ™

Set: "Pull-in" 100%, (for a fraction of a second), then immediately relax only up to 50%, (for only a fraction of a second), and repeat.

Day 5 (**)** *write day*

Assessments: *(circle what applies)*
*Surge Posture: 75% or more of the day / 50% of the day / less than 25% of the day
*Core Posture: 75% or more of the day / 50% of the day / less than 25% of the day
Set Posture: 75% or more of the day / 50% of the day / less than 25% of the day
Breathe Posture: 75% or more of the day / 50% of the day / less than 25% of the day

☐ MORNING: Endurance Technique ™ (1 set), Pulse Technique ™, (1 set), Popins Technique (2 sets).
☐ AFTERNOON: Endurance Technique ™, (after toilet, start of feeding baby, start of changing baby)
☐ BEFORE BED: Endurance ™ (1 set), Pulse ™, (1 set), Popins ™, (in recommended Anti-Gravity Position ™)

Day 6 (**)** *write day*

Assessments: *(circle what applies)*
*Surge Posture: 75% or more of the day / 50% of the day / less than 25% of the day
*Core Posture: 75% or more of the day / 50% of the day / less than 25% of the day
Set Posture: 75% or more of the day / 50% of the day / less than 25% of the day
Breathe Posture: 75% or more of the day / 50% of the day / less than 25% of the day

☐ MORNING: Endurance Technique ™ (1 set), Pulse Technique ™, (1 set), Popins Technique (2 sets).
☐ AFTERNOON: Endurance Technique ™, (after toilet, start of feeding baby, start of changing baby)
☐ BEFORE BED: Endurance ™ (1 set), Pulse ™, (1 set), Popins ™, (in recommended Anti-Gravity Position ™)

Day 7 (**)** *write day*

Assessments: *(circle what applies)*
*Surge Posture: 75% or more of the day / 50% of the day / less than 25% of the day
*Core Posture: 75% or more of the day / 50% of the day / less than 25% of the day
Set Posture: 75% or more of the day / 50% of the day / less than 25% of the day
Breathe Posture: 75% or more of the day / 50% of the day / less than 25% of the day

☐ MORNING: Endurance Technique ™ (1 set), Pulse Technique ™, (1 set), Popins Technique (2 sets).
☐ AFTERNOON: Endurance Technique ™, (after toilet, start of feeding baby, start of changing baby)
☐ BEFORE BED: Endurance ™ (1 set), Pulse ™, (1 set), Popins ™, (in recommended Anti-Gravity Position ™)

Ishio Method ™ Pelvic Floor Rehab (check-off sheet)

Week 10 (/   /20   thru   /   /20   )

Write in your own personal dates.

Adding: **Popins Technique** ™

Set: 10ct / "Pull-in" 100%, (for a fraction of a second), then immediately relax only up to 50%, (for only a fraction of a second), and repeat.

Day 1 (**)** write day

Assessments: (circle what applies)
*Surge Posture: 75% or more of the day / 50% of the day / less than 25% of the day
*Core Posture: 75% or more of the day / 50% of the day / less than 25% of the day
Set Posture: 75% or more of the day / 50% of the day / less than 25% of the day
Breathe Posture: 75% or more of the day / 50% of the day / less than 25% of the day

☐ MORNING: Endurance Technique ™ (1 set), Pulse Technique ™, (1 set), Popins Technique (2 sets).
☐ AFTERNOON: Endurance Technique ™, (after toilet, start of feeding baby, start of changing baby)
☐ BEFORE BED: Endurance ™ (1 set), Pulse ™, (1 set), Popins ™, (in recommended Anti-Gravity Position ™)

Day 2 (**)** write day

Assessments: (circle what applies)
*Surge Posture: 75% or more of the day / 50% of the day / less than 25% of the day
*Core Posture: 75% or more of the day / 50% of the day / less than 25% of the day
Set Posture: 75% or more of the day / 50% of the day / less than 25% of the day
Breathe Posture: 75% or more of the day / 50% of the day / less than 25% of the day

☐ MORNING: Endurance Technique ™ (1 set), Pulse Technique ™, (1 set), Popins Technique (2 sets).
☐ AFTERNOON: Endurance Technique ™, (after toilet, start of feeding baby, start of changing baby)
☐ BEFORE BED: Endurance ™ (1 set), Pulse ™, (1 set), Popins ™, (in recommended Anti-Gravity Position ™)

Day 3 (**)** write day

Assessments: (circle what applies)
*Surge Posture: 75% or more of the day / 50% of the day / less than 25% of the day
*Core Posture: 75% or more of the day / 50% of the day / less than 25% of the day
Set Posture: 75% or more of the day / 50% of the day / less than 25% of the day
Breathe Posture: 75% or more of the day / 50% of the day / less than 25% of the day

☐ MORNING: Endurance Technique ™ (1 set), Pulse Technique ™, (1 set), Popins Technique (2 sets).
☐ AFTERNOON: Endurance Technique ™, (after toilet, start of feeding baby, start of changing baby)
☐ BEFORE BED: Endurance ™ (1 set), Pulse ™, (1 set), Popins ™, (in recommended Anti-Gravity Position ™)

Day 4 (**)** write day

Assessments: (circle what applies)
*Surge Posture: 75% or more of the day / 50% of the day / less than 25% of the day
*Core Posture: 75% or more of the day / 50% of the day / less than 25% of the day
Set Posture: 75% or more of the day / 50% of the day / less than 25% of the day
Breathe Posture: 75% or more of the day / 50% of the day / less than 25% of the day

☐ MORNING: Endurance Technique ™ (1 set), Pulse Technique ™, (1 set), Popins Technique (2 sets).
☐ AFTERNOON: Endurance Technique ™, (after toilet, start of feeding baby, start of changing baby)
☐ BEFORE BED: Endurance ™ (1 set), Pulse ™, (1 set), Popins ™, (in recommended Anti-Gravity Position ™)

Ishio Method ™ Pelvic Floor Rehab (check-off sheet)

Week 10 (/ /20 thru / /20)

Write in your own personal dates.

Adding: Popins Technique ™

Set: 10ct / "Pull-in" 100%, (for a fraction of a second), then immediately relax only up to 50%, (for only a fraction of a second), and repeat.

Day 5 (_____ **)** *write day*

Assessments: *(circle what applies)*
*Surge Posture: 75% or more of the day / 50% of the day / less than 25% of the day
*Core Posture: 75% or more of the day / 50% of the day / less than 25% of the day
Set Posture: 75% or more of the day / 50% of the day / less than 25% of the day
Breathe Posture: 75% or more of the day / 50% of the day / less than 25% of the day

☐ MORNING: Endurance Technique ™ (1 set), Pulse Technique ™, (1 set), Popins Technique (2 sets).
☐ AFTERNOON: Endurance Technique ™, (after toilet, start of feeding baby, start of changing baby)
☐ BEFORE BED: Endurance ™ (1 set), Pulse ™, (1 set), Popins ™, (in recommended Anti-Gravity Position ™)

Day 6 (_____ **)** *write day*

Assessments: *(circle what applies)*
*Surge Posture: 75% or more of the day / 50% of the day / less than 25% of the day
*Core Posture: 75% or more of the day / 50% of the day / less than 25% of the day
Set Posture: 75% or more of the day / 50% of the day / less than 25% of the day
Breathe Posture: 75% or more of the day / 50% of the day / less than 25% of the day

☐ MORNING: Endurance Technique ™ (1 set), Pulse Technique ™, (1 set), Popins Technique (2 sets).
☐ AFTERNOON: Endurance Technique ™, (after toilet, start of feeding baby, start of changing baby)
☐ BEFORE BED: Endurance ™ (1 set), Pulse ™, (1 set), Popins ™, (in recommended Anti-Gravity Position ™)

Day 7 (_____ **)** *write day*

Assessments: *(circle what applies)*
*Surge Posture: 75% or more of the day / 50% of the day / less than 25% of the day
*Core Posture: 75% or more of the day / 50% of the day / less than 25% of the day
Set Posture: 75% or more of the day / 50% of the day / less than 25% of the day
Breathe Posture: 75% or more of the day / 50% of the day / less than 25% of the day

☐ MORNING: Endurance Technique ™ (1 set), Pulse Technique ™, (1 set), Popins Technique (2 sets).
☐ AFTERNOON: Endurance Technique ™, (after toilet, start of feeding baby, start of changing baby)
☐ BEFORE BED: Endurance ™ (1 set), Pulse ™, (1 set), Popins ™, (in recommended Anti-Gravity Position ™)

Ishio Method ™ Pelvic Floor Rehab (check-off sheet)

Week 11 (/   /20   thru   /   /20   ) *Write in your own personal dates.*

Adding: **Iso-Form** ™

Set: Start - Hold for 5 seconds. Goal - increase in increments of 5 seconds, until sets hold for 15 seconds. The goal also is to have fluidity between contracting your VM and your PF Muscles.

Day 1 ( ) *write day*

Assessments: *(circle what applies)*
*Surge Posture: 75% or more of the day / 50% of the day / less than 25% of the day
*Core Posture: 75% or more of the day / 50% of the day / less than 25% of the day
Set Posture: 75% or more of the day / 50% of the day / less than 25% of the day
Breathe Posture: 75% or more of the day / 50% of the day / less than 25% of the day

☐ MORNING: Endurance Tec ™ (1 set), Pulse Tec ™, (1 set), Endurance Tec ™ with Iso-Form ™, (1 set).
☐ AFTERNOON: Endurance Technique ™, (after toilet, start of feeding baby, start of changing baby)
☐ BEFORE BED: Endurance Tec ™ (1 set), Popins Tec ™, (2 sets),Endurance Tec ™ with Iso-Form ™,(2 sets).

Day 2 ( ) *write day*

Assessments: *(circle what applies)*
*Surge Posture: 75% or more of the day / 50% of the day / less than 25% of the day
*Core Posture: 75% or more of the day / 50% of the day / less than 25% of the day
Set Posture: 75% or more of the day / 50% of the day / less than 25% of the day
Breathe Posture: 75% or more of the day / 50% of the day / less than 25% of the day

☐ MORNING: Endurance Tec ™ (1 set), Pulse Tec ™, (1 set), Endurance Tec ™ with Iso-Form ™, (1 set).
☐ AFTERNOON: Endurance Technique ™, (after toilet, start of feeding baby, start of changing baby)
☐ BEFORE BED: Endurance Tec ™ (1 set), Popins Tec ™, (2 sets),Endurance Tec ™ with Iso-Form ™,(2 sets).

Day 3 ( ) *write day*

Assessments: *(circle what applies)*
*Surge Posture: 75% or more of the day / 50% of the day / less than 25% of the day
*Core Posture: 75% or more of the day / 50% of the day / less than 25% of the day
Set Posture: 75% or more of the day / 50% of the day / less than 25% of the day
Breathe Posture: 75% or more of the day / 50% of the day / less than 25% of the day

☐ MORNING: Endurance Tec ™ (1 set), Pulse Tec ™, (1 set), Endurance Tec ™ with Iso-Form ™, (1 set).
☐ AFTERNOON: Endurance Technique ™, (after toilet, start of feeding baby, start of changing baby)
☐ BEFORE BED: Endurance Tec ™ (1 set), Popins Tec ™, (2 sets),Endurance Tec ™ with Iso-Form ™,(2 sets).

Day 4 ( ) *write day*

Assessments: *(circle what applies)*
*Surge Posture: 75% or more of the day / 50% of the day / less than 25% of the day
*Core Posture: 75% or more of the day / 50% of the day / less than 25% of the day
Set Posture: 75% or more of the day / 50% of the day / less than 25% of the day
Breathe Posture: 75% or more of the day / 50% of the day / less than 25% of the day

☐ MORNING: Endurance Tec ™ (1 set), Pulse Tec ™, (1 set), Endurance Tec ™ with Iso-Form ™, (1 set).
☐ AFTERNOON: Endurance Technique ™, (after toilet, start of feeding baby, start of changing baby)
☐ BEFORE BED: Endurance Tec ™ (1 set), Popins Tec ™, (2 sets),Endurance Tec ™ with Iso-Form ™,(2 sets).

Ishio Method ™ Pelvic Floor Rehab (check-off sheet)

Week 11 (/   /20   thru   /   /20   ) *Write in your own personal dates.*

Adding: **Iso-Form** ™

Set: Start - Hold for 5 seconds. Goal - increase in increments of 5 seconds, until sets hold for 15 seconds. The goal also is to have fluidity between contracting your VM and your PF Muscles.

Day 5 (**)** *write day*

Assessments: *(circle what applies)*
*Surge Posture: 75% or more of the day / 50% of the day / less than 25% of the day
*Core Posture: 75% or more of the day / 50% of the day / less than 25% of the day
Set Posture: 75% or more of the day / 50% of the day / less than 25% of the day
Breathe Posture: 75% or more of the day / 50% of the day / less than 25% of the day

☐ MORNING: Endurance Tec ™ (1 set), Pulse Tec ™, (1 set), Endurance Tec ™ with Iso-Form ™, (1 set).
☐ AFTERNOON: Endurance Technique ™, (after toilet, start of feeding baby, start of changing baby)
☐ BEFORE BED: Endurance Tec ™ (1 set), Popins Tec ™, (2 sets),Endurance Tec ™ with Iso-Form ™,(2 sets).

Day 6 (**)** *write day*

Assessments: *(circle what applies)*
*Surge Posture: 75% or more of the day / 50% of the day / less than 25% of the day
*Core Posture: 75% or more of the day / 50% of the day / less than 25% of the day
Set Posture: 75% or more of the day / 50% of the day / less than 25% of the day
Breathe Posture: 75% or more of the day / 50% of the day / less than 25% of the day

☐ MORNING: Endurance Tec ™ (1 set), Pulse Tec ™, (1 set), Endurance Tec ™ with Iso-Form ™, (1 set).
☐ AFTERNOON: Endurance Technique ™, (after toilet, start of feeding baby, start of changing baby)
☐ BEFORE BED: Endurance Tec ™ (1 set), Popins Tec ™, (2 sets),Endurance Tec ™ with Iso-Form ™,(2 sets).

Day 7 (**)** *write day*

Assessments: *(circle what applies)*
*Surge Posture: 75% or more of the day / 50% of the day / less than 25% of the day
*Core Posture: 75% or more of the day / 50% of the day / less than 25% of the day
Set Posture: 75% or more of the day / 50% of the day / less than 25% of the day
Breathe Posture: 75% or more of the day / 50% of the day / less than 25% of the day

☐ MORNING: Endurance Tec ™ (1 set), Pulse Tec ™, (1 set), Endurance Tec ™ with Iso-Form ™, (1 set).
☐ AFTERNOON: Endurance Technique ™, (after toilet, start of feeding baby, start of changing baby)
☐ BEFORE BED: Endurance Tec ™ (1 set), Popins Tec ™, (2 sets),Endurance Tec ™ with Iso-Form ™,(2 sets).

Ishio Method ™ Pelvic Floor Rehab (check-off sheet)

Week 12 (___ / ___ /20   thru   ___ / ___ /20)   *Write in your own personal dates.*

Adding: Iso-Form ™

Set: Start - Hold for 5 seconds. Goal - increase in increments of 5 seconds, until sets hold for 15 seconds. The goal also is to have fluidity between contracting your VM and your PF Muscles.

Day 1 (_____) *write day*

Assessments: *(circle what applies)*
*Surge Posture: 75% or more of the day / 50% of the day / less than 25% of the day
*Core Posture: 75% or more of the day / 50% of the day / less than 25% of the day
Set Posture: 75% or more of the day / 50% of the day / less than 25% of the day
Breathe Posture: 75% or more of the day / 50% of the day / less than 25% of the day

☐ MORNING: Endurance Tec ™ (1 set), Pulse Tec ™, (1 set), Endurance Tec ™ with Iso-Form ™, (1 set).
☐ AFTERNOON: Endurance Technique ™, (after toilet, start of feeding baby, start of changing baby)
☐ BEFORE BED: Endurance Tec ™ (1 set), Popins Tec ™, (2 sets), Endurance Tec ™ with Iso-Form ™, (2 sets).

Day 2 (_____) *write day*

Assessments: *(circle what applies)*
*Surge Posture: 75% or more of the day / 50% of the day / less than 25% of the day
*Core Posture: 75% or more of the day / 50% of the day / less than 25% of the day
Set Posture: 75% or more of the day / 50% of the day / less than 25% of the day
Breathe Posture: 75% or more of the day / 50% of the day / less than 25% of the day

☐ MORNING: Endurance Tec ™ (1 set), Pulse Tec ™, (1 set), Endurance Tec ™ with Iso-Form ™, (1 set).
☐ AFTERNOON: Endurance Technique ™, (after toilet, start of feeding baby, start of changing baby)
☐ BEFORE BED: Endurance Tec ™ (1 set), Popins Tec ™, (2 sets), Endurance Tec ™ with Iso-Form ™, (2 sets).

Day 3 (_____) *write day*

Assessments: *(circle what applies)*
*Surge Posture: 75% or more of the day / 50% of the day / less than 25% of the day
*Core Posture: 75% or more of the day / 50% of the day / less than 25% of the day
Set Posture: 75% or more of the day / 50% of the day / less than 25% of the day
Breathe Posture: 75% or more of the day / 50% of the day / less than 25% of the day

☐ MORNING: Endurance Tec ™ (1 set), Pulse Tec ™, (1 set), Endurance Tec ™ with Iso-Form ™, (1 set).
☐ AFTERNOON: Endurance Technique ™, (after toilet, start of feeding baby, start of changing baby)
☐ BEFORE BED: Endurance Tec ™ (1 set), Popins Tec ™, (2 sets), Endurance Tec ™ with Iso-Form ™, (2 sets).

Day 4 (_____) *write day*

Assessments: *(circle what applies)*
*Surge Posture: 75% or more of the day / 50% of the day / less than 25% of the day
*Core Posture: 75% or more of the day / 50% of the day / less than 25% of the day
Set Posture: 75% or more of the day / 50% of the day / less than 25% of the day
Breathe Posture: 75% or more of the day / 50% of the day / less than 25% of the day

☐ MORNING: Endurance Tec ™ (1 set), Pulse Tec ™, (1 set), Endurance Tec ™ with Iso-Form ™, (1 set).
☐ AFTERNOON: Endurance Technique ™, (after toilet, start of feeding baby, start of changing baby)
☐ BEFORE BED: Endurance Tec ™ (1 set), Popins Tec ™, (2 sets), Endurance Tec ™ with Iso-Form ™, (2 sets).

Ishio Method ™ Pelvic Floor Rehab (check-off sheet)

Week 12 (/   /20   thru   /   /20   )   *Write in your own personal dates.*

Adding: **Iso-Form** ™

Set: Start - Hold for 5 seconds. Goal - increase in increments of 5 seconds, until sets hold for 15 seconds. The goal also is to have fluidity between contracting your VM and your PF Muscles.

Day 5 (_____ **)** *write day*

Assessments: *(circle what applies)*
*Surge Posture: 75% or more of the day / 50% of the day / less than 25% of the day
*Core Posture: 75% or more of the day / 50% of the day / less than 25% of the day
Set Posture: 75% or more of the day / 50% of the day / less than 25% of the day
Breathe Posture: 75% or more of the day / 50% of the day / less than 25% of the day

- ☐ MORNING: Endurance Tec ™ (1 set), Pulse Tec ™, (1 set), Endurance Tec ™ with Iso-Form ™, (1 set).
- ☐ AFTERNOON: Endurance Technique ™, (after toilet, start of feeding baby, start of changing baby)
- ☐ BEFORE BED: Endurance Tec ™ (1 set), Popins Tec ™, (2 sets),Endurance Tec ™ with Iso-Form ™,(2 sets).

Day 6 (_____ **)** *write day*

Assessments: *(circle what applies)*
*Surge Posture: 75% or more of the day / 50% of the day / less than 25% of the day
*Core Posture: 75% or more of the day / 50% of the day / less than 25% of the day
Set Posture: 75% or more of the day / 50% of the day / less than 25% of the day
Breathe Posture: 75% or more of the day / 50% of the day / less than 25% of the day

- ☐ MORNING: Endurance Tec ™ (1 set), Pulse Tec ™, (1 set), Endurance Tec ™ with Iso-Form ™, (1 set).
- ☐ AFTERNOON: Endurance Technique ™, (after toilet, start of feeding baby, start of changing baby)
- ☐ BEFORE BED: Endurance Tec ™ (1 set), Popins Tec ™, (2 sets),Endurance Tec ™ with Iso-Form ™,(2 sets).

Day 7 (_____ **)** *write day*

Assessments: *(circle what applies)*
*Surge Posture: 75% or more of the day / 50% of the day / less than 25% of the day
*Core Posture: 75% or more of the day / 50% of the day / less than 25% of the day
Set Posture: 75% or more of the day / 50% of the day / less than 25% of the day
Breathe Posture: 75% or more of the day / 50% of the day / less than 25% of the day

- ☐ MORNING: Endurance Tec ™ (1 set), Pulse Tec ™, (1 set), Endurance Tec ™ with Iso-Form ™, (1 set).
- ☐ AFTERNOON: Endurance Technique ™, (after toilet, start of feeding baby, start of changing baby)
- ☐ BEFORE BED: Endurance Tec ™ (1 set), Popins Tec ™, (2 sets),Endurance Tec ™ with Iso-Form ™,(2 sets).

Ishio Method ™ Pelvic Floor Rehab (check-off sheet)

Week 13 (/   /20   thru   /   /20   )

Write in your own personal dates.

Adding: **Iso-Form** ™

Set: Start - Hold for 5 seconds. Goal - increase in increments of 5 seconds, until sets hold for 15 seconds. The goal also is to have fluidity between contracting your VM and your PF Muscles.

Day 1 (**)** *write day*

Assessments: *(circle what applies)*
*Surge Posture: 75% or more of the day / 50% of the day / less than 25% of the day
*Core Posture: 75% or more of the day / 50% of the day / less than 25% of the day
Set Posture: 75% or more of the day / 50% of the day / less than 25% of the day
Breathe Posture: 75% or more of the day / 50% of the day / less than 25% of the day

☐ MORNING: Endurance Tec ™ (1 set), Pulse Tec ™, (1 set), Endurance Tec ™ with Iso-Form ™, (1 set).
☐ AFTERNOON: Endurance Technique ™, (after toilet, start of feeding baby, start of changing baby)
☐ BEFORE BED: Endurance Tec ™ (1 set), Popins Tec ™, (2 sets),Endurance Tec ™ with Iso-Form ™,(2 sets).

Day 2 (**)** *write day*

Assessments: *(circle what applies)*
*Surge Posture: 75% or more of the day / 50% of the day / less than 25% of the day
*Core Posture: 75% or more of the day / 50% of the day / less than 25% of the day
Set Posture: 75% or more of the day / 50% of the day / less than 25% of the day
Breathe Posture: 75% or more of the day / 50% of the day / less than 25% of the day

☐ MORNING: Endurance Tec ™ (1 set), Pulse Tec ™, (1 set), Endurance Tec ™ with Iso-Form ™, (1 set).
☐ AFTERNOON: Endurance Technique ™, (after toilet, start of feeding baby, start of changing baby)
☐ BEFORE BED: Endurance Tec ™ (1 set), Popins Tec ™, (2 sets),Endurance Tec ™ with Iso-Form ™,(2 sets).

Day 3 (**)** *write day*

Assessments: *(circle what applies)*
*Surge Posture: 75% or more of the day / 50% of the day / less than 25% of the day
*Core Posture: 75% or more of the day / 50% of the day / less than 25% of the day
Set Posture: 75% or more of the day / 50% of the day / less than 25% of the day
Breathe Posture: 75% or more of the day / 50% of the day / less than 25% of the day

☐ MORNING: Endurance Tec ™ (1 set), Pulse Tec ™, (1 set), Endurance Tec ™ with Iso-Form ™, (1 set).
☐ AFTERNOON: Endurance Technique ™, (after toilet, start of feeding baby, start of changing baby)
☐ BEFORE BED: Endurance Tec ™ (1 set), Popins Tec ™, (2 sets),Endurance Tec ™ with Iso-Form ™,(2 sets).

Day 4 (**)** *write day*

Assessments: *(circle what applies)*
*Surge Posture: 75% or more of the day / 50% of the day / less than 25% of the day
*Core Posture: 75% or more of the day / 50% of the day / less than 25% of the day
Set Posture: 75% or more of the day / 50% of the day / less than 25% of the day
Breathe Posture: 75% or more of the day / 50% of the day / less than 25% of the day

☐ MORNING: Endurance Tec ™ (1 set), Pulse Tec ™, (1 set), Endurance Tec ™ with Iso-Form ™, (1 set).
☐ AFTERNOON: Endurance Technique ™, (after toilet, start of feeding baby, start of changing baby)
☐ BEFORE BED: Endurance Tec ™ (1 set), Popins Tec ™, (2 sets),Endurance Tec ™ with Iso-Form ™,(2 sets).

Ishio Method ™ Pelvic Floor Rehab (check-off sheet)

Week 13   (/   /20   thru   /   /20   )

Write in your own personal dates.

Adding: Iso-Form ™

Set: Start - Hold for 5 seconds. Goal - increase in increments of 5 seconds, until sets hold for 15 seconds. The goal also is to have fluidity between contracting your VM and your PF Muscles.

Day 5 (_____ **)** *write day*

Assessments: *(circle what applies)*
*Surge Posture: 75% or more of the day / 50% of the day / less than 25% of the day
*Core Posture: 75% or more of the day / 50% of the day / less than 25% of the day
Set Posture: 75% or more of the day / 50% of the day / less than 25% of the day
Breathe Posture: 75% or more of the day / 50% of the day / less than 25% of the day

☐ MORNING: Endurance Tec ™ (1 set), Pulse Tec ™, (1 set), Endurance Tec ™ with Iso-Form ™, (1 set).
☐ AFTERNOON: Endurance Technique ™, (after toilet, start of feeding baby, start of changing baby)
☐ BEFORE BED: Endurance Tec ™ (1 set), Popins Tec ™, (2 sets),Endurance Tec ™ with Iso-Form ™,(2 sets).

Day 6 (_____ **)** *write day*

Assessments: *(circle what applies)*
*Surge Posture: 75% or more of the day / 50% of the day / less than 25% of the day
*Core Posture: 75% or more of the day / 50% of the day / less than 25% of the day
Set Posture: 75% or more of the day / 50% of the day / less than 25% of the day
Breathe Posture: 75% or more of the day / 50% of the day / less than 25% of the day

☐ MORNING: Endurance Tec ™ (1 set), Pulse Tec ™, (1 set), Endurance Tec ™ with Iso-Form ™, (1 set).
☐ AFTERNOON: Endurance Technique ™, (after toilet, start of feeding baby, start of changing baby)
☐ BEFORE BED: Endurance Tec ™ (1 set), Popins Tec ™, (2 sets),Endurance Tec ™ with Iso-Form ™,(2 sets).

Day 7 (_____ **)** *write day*

Assessments: *(circle what applies)*
*Surge Posture: 75% or more of the day / 50% of the day / less than 25% of the day
*Core Posture: 75% or more of the day / 50% of the day / less than 25% of the day
Set Posture: 75% or more of the day / 50% of the day / less than 25% of the day
Breathe Posture: 75% or more of the day / 50% of the day / less than 25% of the day

☐ MORNING: Endurance Tec ™ (1 set), Pulse Tec ™, (1 set), Endurance Tec ™ with Iso-Form ™, (1 set).
☐ AFTERNOON: Endurance Technique ™, (after toilet, start of feeding baby, start of changing baby)
☐ BEFORE BED: Endurance Tec ™ (1 set), Popins Tec ™, (2 sets),Endurance Tec ™ with Iso-Form ™,(2 sets).

Ishio Method ™ Pelvic Floor Rehab (check-off sheet)

Week 14 (/   /20   thru   /   /20   )

Write in your own personal dates.

Adding: Iso-Form ™

Set: Start - Hold for 5 seconds. Goal - increase in increments of 5 seconds, until sets hold for 15 seconds. The goal also is to have fluidity between contracting your VM and your PF Muscles.

Day 1 (**)** *write day*

Assessments: *(circle what applies)*
*Surge Posture: 75% or more of the day / 50% of the day / less than 25% of the day
*Core Posture: 75% or more of the day / 50% of the day / less than 25% of the day
Set Posture: 75% or more of the day / 50% of the day / less than 25% of the day
Breathe Posture: 75% or more of the day / 50% of the day / less than 25% of the day

☐ MORNING: Endurance Tec ™ (1 set), Pulse Tec ™, (1 set), Endurance Tec ™ with Iso-Form ™, (1 set).
☐ AFTERNOON: Endurance Technique ™, (after toilet, start of feeding baby, start of changing baby)
☐ BEFORE BED: Endurance Tec ™ (1 set), Popins Tec ™, (2 sets), Endurance Tec ™ with Iso-Form ™, (2 sets).

Day 2 (**)** *write day*

Assessments: *(circle what applies)*
*Surge Posture: 75% or more of the day / 50% of the day / less than 25% of the day
*Core Posture: 75% or more of the day / 50% of the day / less than 25% of the day
Set Posture: 75% or more of the day / 50% of the day / less than 25% of the day
Breathe Posture: 75% or more of the day / 50% of the day / less than 25% of the day

☐ MORNING: Endurance Tec ™ (1 set), Pulse Tec ™, (1 set), Endurance Tec ™ with Iso-Form ™, (1 set).
☐ AFTERNOON: Endurance Technique ™, (after toilet, start of feeding baby, start of changing baby)
☐ BEFORE BED: Endurance Tec ™ (1 set), Popins Tec ™, (2 sets), Endurance Tec ™ with Iso-Form ™, (2 sets).

Day 3 (**)** *write day*

Assessments: *(circle what applies)*
*Surge Posture: 75% or more of the day / 50% of the day / less than 25% of the day
*Core Posture: 75% or more of the day / 50% of the day / less than 25% of the day
Set Posture: 75% or more of the day / 50% of the day / less than 25% of the day
Breathe Posture: 75% or more of the day / 50% of the day / less than 25% of the day

☐ MORNING: Endurance Tec ™ (1 set), Pulse Tec ™, (1 set), Endurance Tec ™ with Iso-Form ™, (1 set).
☐ AFTERNOON: Endurance Technique ™, (after toilet, start of feeding baby, start of changing baby)
☐ BEFORE BED: Endurance Tec ™ (1 set), Popins Tec ™, (2 sets), Endurance Tec ™ with Iso-Form ™, (2 sets).

Day 4 (**)** *write day*

Assessments: *(circle what applies)*
*Surge Posture: 75% or more of the day / 50% of the day / less than 25% of the day
*Core Posture: 75% or more of the day / 50% of the day / less than 25% of the day
Set Posture: 75% or more of the day / 50% of the day / less than 25% of the day
Breathe Posture: 75% or more of the day / 50% of the day / less than 25% of the day

☐ MORNING: Endurance Tec ™ (1 set), Pulse Tec ™, (1 set), Endurance Tec ™ with Iso-Form ™, (1 set).
☐ AFTERNOON: Endurance Technique ™, (after toilet, start of feeding baby, start of changing baby)
☐ BEFORE BED: Endurance Tec ™ (1 set), Popins Tec ™, (2 sets), Endurance Tec ™ with Iso-Form ™, (2 sets).

Ishio Method ™ Pelvic Floor Rehab (check-off sheet)

Week 14 (/   /20   thru   /   /20   )

Write in your own personal dates.

Adding: **Iso-Form** ™

Set: Start - Hold for 5 seconds. Goal - increase in increments of 5 seconds, until sets hold for 15 seconds. The goal also is to have fluidity between contracting your VM and your PF Muscles.

Day 5 (**)** *write day*

Assessments: *(circle what applies)*
*Surge Posture: 75% or more of the day / 50% of the day / less than 25% of the day
*Core Posture: 75% or more of the day / 50% of the day / less than 25% of the day
Set Posture: 75% or more of the day / 50% of the day / less than 25% of the day
Breathe Posture: 75% or more of the day / 50% of the day / less than 25% of the day

☐ MORNING: Endurance Tec ™ (1 set), Pulse Tec ™, (1 set), Endurance Tec ™ with Iso-Form ™, (1 set).
☐ AFTERNOON: Endurance Technique ™, (after toilet, start of feeding baby, start of changing baby)
☐ BEFORE BED: Endurance Tec ™ (1 set), Popins Tec ™, (2 sets),Endurance Tec ™ with Iso-Form ™,(2 sets).

Day 6 (**)** *write day*

Assessments: *(circle what applies)*
*Surge Posture: 75% or more of the day / 50% of the day / less than 25% of the day
*Core Posture: 75% or more of the day / 50% of the day / less than 25% of the day
Set Posture: 75% or more of the day / 50% of the day / less than 25% of the day
Breathe Posture: 75% or more of the day / 50% of the day / less than 25% of the day

☐ MORNING: Endurance Tec ™ (1 set), Pulse Tec ™, (1 set), Endurance Tec ™ with Iso-Form ™, (1 set).
☐ AFTERNOON: Endurance Technique ™, (after toilet, start of feeding baby, start of changing baby)
☐ BEFORE BED: Endurance Tec ™ (1 set), Popins Tec ™, (2 sets),Endurance Tec ™ with Iso-Form ™,(2 sets).

Day 7 (**)** *write day*

Assessments: *(circle what applies)*
*Surge Posture: 75% or more of the day / 50% of the day / less than 25% of the day
*Core Posture: 75% or more of the day / 50% of the day / less than 25% of the day
Set Posture: 75% or more of the day / 50% of the day / less than 25% of the day
Breathe Posture: 75% or more of the day / 50% of the day / less than 25% of the day

☐ MORNING: Endurance Tec ™ (1 set), Pulse Tec ™, (1 set), Endurance Tec ™ with Iso-Form ™, (1 set).
☐ AFTERNOON: Endurance Technique ™, (after toilet, start of feeding baby, start of changing baby)
☐ BEFORE BED: Endurance Tec ™ (1 set), Popins Tec ™, (2 sets),Endurance Tec ™ with Iso-Form ™,(2 sets).

Ishio Method ™ Pelvic Floor Rehab (check-off sheet)

Week 15 (/   /20   thru   /   /20   ) *Write in your own personal dates.*

Adding: **Pulse Technique** ™ **WITH Iso-Form** ™

Day 1 ( ) *write day*

Assessments: *(circle what applies)*
*Surge Posture: 75% or more of the day / 50% of the day / less than 25% of the day
*Core Posture: 75% or more of the day / 50% of the day / less than 25% of the day
Set Posture: 75% or more of the day / 50% of the day / less than 25% of the day
Breathe Posture: 75% or more of the day / 50% of the day / less than 25% of the day

☐ MORNING: Popins Tech ™ (2 sets) / WITH Iso-Form ™ - Endurance Tech ™ (1 set)
☐ AFTERNOON: Endurance Technique ™, (after toilet, start of feeding baby, start of changing baby)
☐ BEFORE BED: Endurance Tec ™ (1 set) / WITH Iso-Form ™ Pulse Tech ™ (2 sets)

Day 2 ( ) *write day*

Assessments: *(circle what applies)*
*Surge Posture: 75% or more of the day / 50% of the day / less than 25% of the day
*Core Posture: 75% or more of the day / 50% of the day / less than 25% of the day
Set Posture: 75% or more of the day / 50% of the day / less than 25% of the day
Breathe Posture: 75% or more of the day / 50% of the day / less than 25% of the day

☐ MORNING: Popins Tech ™ (2 sets) / WITH Iso-Form ™ - Endurance Tech ™ (1 set)
☐ AFTERNOON: Endurance Technique ™, (after toilet, start of feeding baby, start of changing baby)
☐ BEFORE BED: Endurance Tec ™ (1 set) / WITH Iso-Form ™ Pulse Tech ™ (2 sets)

Day 3 ( ) *write day*

Assessments: *(circle what applies)*
*Surge Posture: 75% or more of the day / 50% of the day / less than 25% of the day
*Core Posture: 75% or more of the day / 50% of the day / less than 25% of the day
Set Posture: 75% or more of the day / 50% of the day / less than 25% of the day
Breathe Posture: 75% or more of the day / 50% of the day / less than 25% of the day

☐ MORNING: Popins Tech ™ (2 sets) / WITH Iso-Form ™ - Endurance Tech ™ (1 set)
☐ AFTERNOON: Endurance Technique ™, (after toilet, start of feeding baby, start of changing baby)
☐ BEFORE BED: Endurance Tec ™ (1 set) / WITH Iso-Form ™ Pulse Tech ™ (2 sets)

Day 4 ( ) *write day*

Assessments: *(circle what applies)*
*Surge Posture: 75% or more of the day / 50% of the day / less than 25% of the day
*Core Posture: 75% or more of the day / 50% of the day / less than 25% of the day
Set Posture: 75% or more of the day / 50% of the day / less than 25% of the day
Breathe Posture: 75% or more of the day / 50% of the day / less than 25% of the day

☐ MORNING: Popins Tech ™ (2 sets) / WITH Iso-Form ™ - Endurance Tech ™ (1 set)
☐ AFTERNOON: Endurance Technique ™, (after toilet, start of feeding baby, start of changing baby)
☐ BEFORE BED: Endurance Tec ™ (1 set) / WITH Iso-Form ™ Pulse Tech ™ (2 sets)

Ishio Method ™ Pelvic Floor Rehab (check-off sheet)
Week 15 (/ /20 thru / /20) *Write in your own personal dates.*
Adding: **Pulse Technique ™ WITH Iso-Form ™**

Day 5 ( ) *write day*

Assessments: *(circle what applies)*
*Surge Posture: 75% or more of the day / 50% of the day / less than 25% of the day
*Core Posture: 75% or more of the day / 50% of the day / less than 25% of the day
Set Posture: 75% or more of the day / 50% of the day / less than 25% of the day
Breathe Posture: 75% or more of the day / 50% of the day / less than 25% of the day

☐ MORNING: Popins Tech ™ (2 sets) / WITH Iso-Form ™ - Endurance Tech ™ (1 set) & Pulse Tech ™, (1 set).
☐ AFTERNOON: Endurance Technique ™, (after toilet, start of feeding baby, start of changing baby)
☐ BEFORE BED: Endurance Tec ™ (1 set) / WITH Iso-Form ™ - Endurance Tec ™ (1 set) & Pulse Tec ™ (2 sets)

Day 6 ( ) *write day*

Assessments: *(circle what applies)*
*Surge Posture: 75% or more of the day / 50% of the day / less than 25% of the day
*Core Posture: 75% or more of the day / 50% of the day / less than 25% of the day
Set Posture: 75% or more of the day / 50% of the day / less than 25% of the day
Breathe Posture: 75% or more of the day / 50% of the day / less than 25% of the day

☐ MORNING: Popins Tech ™ (2 sets) / WITH Iso-Form ™ - Endurance Tech ™ (1 set) & Pulse Tech ™, (1 set).
☐ AFTERNOON: Endurance Technique ™, (after toilet, start of feeding baby, start of changing baby)
☐ BEFORE BED: Endurance Tec ™ (1 set) / WITH Iso-Form ™ - Endurance Tec ™ (1 set) & Pulse Tec ™ (2 sets)

Day 7 ( ) *write day*

Assessments: *(circle what applies)*
*Surge Posture: 75% or more of the day / 50% of the day / less than 25% of the day
*Core Posture: 75% or more of the day / 50% of the day / less than 25% of the day
Set Posture: 75% or more of the day / 50% of the day / less than 25% of the day
Breathe Posture: 75% or more of the day / 50% of the day / less than 25% of the day

☐ MORNING: Popins Tech ™ (2 sets) / WITH Iso-Form ™ - Endurance Tech ™ (1 set) & Pulse Tech ™, (1 set).
☐ AFTERNOON: Endurance Technique ™, (after toilet, start of feeding baby, start of changing baby)
☐ BEFORE BED: Endurance Tec ™ (1 set) / WITH Iso-Form ™ - Endurance Tec ™ (1 set) & Pulse Tec ™ (2 sets)

Ishio Method ™ Pelvic Floor Rehab (check-off sheet)

Week 16 (/   /20   thru   /   /20   ) *Write in your own personal dates.*

Adding: **Pulse Technique** ™ <u>**WITH**</u> **Iso-Form** ™

Day 1 (**)** *write day*

Assessments: *(circle what applies)*
*<u>Surge Posture</u>: 75% or more of the day / 50% of the day / less than 25% of the day
*<u>Core Posture</u>: 75% or more of the day / 50% of the day / less than 25% of the day
<u>Set Posture</u>: 75% or more of the day / 50% of the day / less than 25% of the day
<u>Breathe Posture</u>: 75% or more of the day / 50% of the day / less than 25% of the day

☐ MORNING: Popins Tech ™ (2 sets) / WITH Iso-Form ™ - Endurance Tech ™ (1 set)
☐ AFTERNOON: Endurance Technique ™, (after toilet, start of feeding baby, start of changing baby)
☐ BEFORE BED: Endurance Tec ™ (1 set) / WITH Iso-Form ™ Pulse Tech ™ (2 sets)

Day 2 (**)** *write day*

Assessments: *(circle what applies)*
*<u>Surge Posture</u>: 75% or more of the day / 50% of the day / less than 25% of the day
*<u>Core Posture</u>: 75% or more of the day / 50% of the day / less than 25% of the day
<u>Set Posture</u>: 75% or more of the day / 50% of the day / less than 25% of the day
<u>Breathe Posture</u>: 75% or more of the day / 50% of the day / less than 25% of the day

☐ MORNING: Popins Tech ™ (2 sets) / WITH Iso-Form ™ - Endurance Tech ™ (1 set)
☐ AFTERNOON: Endurance Technique ™, (after toilet, start of feeding baby, start of changing baby)
☐ BEFORE BED: Endurance Tec ™ (1 set) / WITH Iso-Form ™ Pulse Tech ™ (2 sets)

Day 3 (**)** *write day*

Assessments: *(circle what applies)*
*<u>Surge Posture</u>: 75% or more of the day / 50% of the day / less than 25% of the day
*<u>Core Posture</u>: 75% or more of the day / 50% of the day / less than 25% of the day
<u>Set Posture</u>: 75% or more of the day / 50% of the day / less than 25% of the day
<u>Breathe Posture</u>: 75% or more of the day / 50% of the day / less than 25% of the day

☐ MORNING: Popins Tech ™ (2 sets) / WITH Iso-Form ™ - Endurance Tech ™ (1 set)
☐ AFTERNOON: Endurance Technique ™, (after toilet, start of feeding baby, start of changing baby)
☐ BEFORE BED: Endurance Tec ™ (1 set) / WITH Iso-Form ™ Pulse Tech ™ (2 sets)

Day 4 (**)** *write day*

Assessments: *(circle what applies)*
*<u>Surge Posture</u>: 75% or more of the day / 50% of the day / less than 25% of the day
*<u>Core Posture</u>: 75% or more of the day / 50% of the day / less than 25% of the day
<u>Set Posture</u>: 75% or more of the day / 50% of the day / less than 25% of the day
<u>Breathe Posture</u>: 75% or more of the day / 50% of the day / less than 25% of the day

☐ MORNING: Popins Tech ™ (2 sets) / WITH Iso-Form ™ - Endurance Tech ™ (1 set)
☐ AFTERNOON: Endurance Technique ™, (after toilet, start of feeding baby, start of changing baby)
☐ BEFORE BED: Endurance Tec ™ (1 set) / WITH Iso-Form ™ Pulse Tech ™ (2 sets)

Ishio Method ™ Pelvic Floor Rehab (check-off sheet)

Week 16 (/ /20 thru / /20) *Write in your own personal dates.*

Adding: **Pulse Technique ™ WITH Iso-Form ™**

Day 5 ( ) *write day*

Assessments: *(circle what applies)*
*Surge Posture: 75% or more of the day / 50% of the day / less than 25% of the day
*Core Posture: 75% or more of the day / 50% of the day / less than 25% of the day
Set Posture: 75% or more of the day / 50% of the day / less than 25% of the day
Breathe Posture: 75% or more of the day / 50% of the day / less than 25% of the day

☐ MORNING: Popins Tech ™ (2 sets) / WITH Iso-Form ™ - Endurance Tech ™ (1 set)
☐ AFTERNOON: Endurance Technique ™, (after toilet, start of feeding baby, start of changing baby)
☐ BEFORE BED: Endurance Tec ™ (1 set) / WITH Iso-Form ™ Pulse Tech ™ (2 sets)

Day 6 ( ) *write day*

Assessments: *(circle what applies)*
*Surge Posture: 75% or more of the day / 50% of the day / less than 25% of the day
*Core Posture: 75% or more of the day / 50% of the day / less than 25% of the day
Set Posture: 75% or more of the day / 50% of the day / less than 25% of the day
Breathe Posture: 75% or more of the day / 50% of the day / less than 25% of the day

☐ MORNING: Popins Tech ™ (2 sets) / WITH Iso-Form ™ - Endurance Tech ™ (1 set)
☐ AFTERNOON: Endurance Technique ™, (after toilet, start of feeding baby, start of changing baby)
☐ BEFORE BED: Endurance Tec ™ (1 set) / WITH Iso-Form ™ Pulse Tech ™ (2 sets)

Day 7 ( ) *write day*

Assessments: *(circle what applies)*
*Surge Posture: 75% or more of the day / 50% of the day / less than 25% of the day
*Core Posture: 75% or more of the day / 50% of the day / less than 25% of the day
Set Posture: 75% or more of the day / 50% of the day / less than 25% of the day
Breathe Posture: 75% or more of the day / 50% of the day / less than 25% of the day

☐ MORNING: Popins Tech ™ (2 sets) / WITH Iso-Form ™ - Endurance Tech ™ (1 set)
☐ AFTERNOON: Endurance Technique ™, (after toilet, start of feeding baby, start of changing baby)
☐ BEFORE BED: Endurance Tec ™ (1 set) / WITH Iso-Form ™ Pulse Tech ™ (2 sets)

Ishio Method ™ Abdominal Rehab (check-off sheet)

Week 1 (/   /20   thru   /   /20   )

Write in your own personal dates.

Ishio Method - Post Pregnancy Key Principles ™

Get Acquainted: Core Posture ™, Surge Posture ™, Set Posture ™, Breathe Posture ™

Day 1 ( ) *write day*

Practice: *(circle what applies)*

*Surge Posture: 75% or more of the day / 50% of the day / less than 25% of the day
*Core Posture: 75% or more of the day / 50% of the day / less than 25% of the day
Set Posture: 75% or more of the day / 50% of the day / less than 25% of the day
Breathe Posture: 75% or more of the day / 50% of the day / less than 25% of the day

Wear your Sillo Belly Wrap ™, (more than half the day, and at night):
75% or more of the day / 50% of the day / less than 25% of the day

---

Day 2 ( ) *write day*

Practice: *(circle what applies)*

*Surge Posture: 75% or more of the day / 50% of the day / less than 25% of the day
*Core Posture: 75% or more of the day / 50% of the day / less than 25% of the day
Set Posture: 75% or more of the day / 50% of the day / less than 25% of the day
Breathe Posture: 75% or more of the day / 50% of the day / less than 25% of the day

Wear your Sillo Belly Wrap ™, (more than half the day, and at night):
75% or more of the day / 50% of the day / less than 25% of the day

---

Day 3 ( ) *write day*

Practice: *(circle what applies)*

*Surge Posture: 75% or more of the day / 50% of the day / less than 25% of the day
*Core Posture: 75% or more of the day / 50% of the day / less than 25% of the day
Set Posture: 75% or more of the day / 50% of the day / less than 25% of the day
Breathe Posture: 75% or more of the day / 50% of the day / less than 25% of the day

Wear your Sillo Belly Wrap ™, (more than half the day, and at night):
75% or more of the day / 50% of the day / less than 25% of the day

---

Day 4 ( ) *write day*

Practice: *(circle what applies)*

*Surge Posture: 75% or more of the day / 50% of the day / less than 25% of the day
*Core Posture: 75% or more of the day / 50% of the day / less than 25% of the day
Set Posture: 75% or more of the day / 50% of the day / less than 25% of the day
Breathe Posture: 75% or more of the day / 50% of the day / less than 25% of the day

Wear your Sillo Belly Wrap ™, (more than half the day, and at night):
75% or more of the day / 50% of the day / less than 25% of the day

Ishio Method ™ Abdominal Rehab (check-off sheet)

Week 1 (/   /20   thru   /   /20   )

Write in your own personal dates.

Ishio Method - Post Pregnancy Key Principles ™

Get Acquainted: Core Posture ™, Surge Posture ™, Set Posture ™, Breathe Posture ™

Day 5 (   ) *write day*

Practice: *(circle what applies)*

*Surge Posture: 75% or more of the day / 50% of the day / less than 25% of the day
*Core Posture: 75% or more of the day / 50% of the day / less than 25% of the day
Set Posture: 75% or more of the day / 50% of the day / less than 25% of the day
Breathe Posture: 75% or more of the day / 50% of the day / less than 25% of the day

Wear your Sillo Belly Wrap ™, (more than half the day, and at night):
75% or more of the day / 50% of the day / less than 25% of the day

Day 6 (   ) *write day*

Practice: *(circle what applies)*

*Surge Posture: 75% or more of the day / 50% of the day / less than 25% of the day
*Core Posture: 75% or more of the day / 50% of the day / less than 25% of the day
Set Posture: 75% or more of the day / 50% of the day / less than 25% of the day
Breathe Posture: 75% or more of the day / 50% of the day / less than 25% of the day

Wear your Sillo Belly Wrap ™, (more than half the day, and at night):
75% or more of the day / 50% of the day / less than 25% of the day

Day 7 (   ) *write day*

Practice: *(circle what applies)*

*Surge Posture: 75% or more of the day / 50% of the day / less than 25% of the day
*Core Posture: 75% or more of the day / 50% of the day / less than 25% of the day
Set Posture: 75% or more of the day / 50% of the day / less than 25% of the day
Breathe Posture: 75% or more of the day / 50% of the day / less than 25% of the day

Wear your Sillo Belly Wrap ™, (more than half the day, and at night):
75% or more of the day / 50% of the day / less than 25% of the day

Ishio Method ™ Abdominal Rehab (check-off sheet)

Week 2 (/   /20   thru   /   /20   )

Write in your own personal dates.

Seated Pull-ins ™

Rep: 7 reps per set. Breathe in, (allowing your abs to relax), then as you breathe out, pull-in your abs as far in as possible)

Day 1 (_____ **)** *write day*

> **Important:** Wear your Sillo Belly Wrap ™ every night, (crossing in the front).

Assessments: *(circle what applies)*
*Surge Posture: 75% or more of the day / 50% of the day / less than 25% of the day
*Core Posture: 75% or more of the day / 50% of the day / less than 25% of the day
Set Posture: 75% or more of the day / 50% of the day / less than 25% of the day
Breathe Posture: 75% or more of the day / 50% of the day / less than 25% of the day

☐ Morning meal
☐ Afternoon meal
☐ Evening meal

☐ _____ (fill-in when you did exercise,
☐ _____ example, standing in line, etc)
☐ _____

Day 2 (_____ **)** *write day*

Assessments: *(circle what applies)*
*Surge Posture: 75% or more of the day / 50% of the day / less than 25% of the day
*Core Posture: 75% or more of the day / 50% of the day / less than 25% of the day
Set Posture: 75% or more of the day / 50% of the day / less than 25% of the day
Breathe Posture: 75% or more of the day / 50% of the day / less than 25% of the day

☐ Morning meal
☐ Afternoon meal
☐ Evening meal

☐ _____ (fill-in when you did exercise,
☐ _____ example, standing in line, etc)
☐ _____

Day 3 (_____ **)** *write day*

Assessments: *(circle what applies)*
*Surge Posture: 75% or more of the day / 50% of the day / less than 25% of the day
*Core Posture: 75% or more of the day / 50% of the day / less than 25% of the day
Set Posture: 75% or more of the day / 50% of the day / less than 25% of the day
Breathe Posture: 75% or more of the day / 50% of the day / less than 25% of the day

☐ Morning meal
☐ Afternoon meal
☐ Evening meal

☐ _____ (fill-in when you did exercise,
☐ _____ example, standing in line, etc)
☐ _____

Day 4 (_____ **)** *write day*

Assessments: *(circle what applies)*
*Surge Posture: 75% or more of the day / 50% of the day / less than 25% of the day
*Core Posture: 75% or more of the day / 50% of the day / less than 25% of the day
Set Posture: 75% or more of the day / 50% of the day / less than 25% of the day
Breathe Posture: 75% or more of the day / 50% of the day / less than 25% of the day

☐ Morning meal
☐ Afternoon meal
☐ Evening meal

☐ _____ (fill-in when you did exercise,
☐ _____ example, standing in line, etc)
☐ _____

Ishio Method ™ Abdominal Rehab (check-off sheet)

Week 2 (/   /20   thru   /   /20   )

Write in your own personal dates.

Seated Pull-ins ™

Rep: 7 reps per set. Breathe in, (allowing your abs to relax), then as you breathe out, pull-in your abs as far in as possible)

Day 5 (_____ **)** *write day*

| **Important:** Wear your Sillo Belly Wrap ™ every night, (crossing in the front). |

Assessments: *(circle what applies)*
*Surge Posture: 75% or more of the day / 50% of the day / less than 25% of the day
*Core Posture: 75% or more of the day / 50% of the day / less than 25% of the day
Set Posture: 75% or more of the day / 50% of the day / less than 25% of the day
Breathe Posture: 75% or more of the day / 50% of the day / less than 25% of the day

- ☐ Morning meal
- ☐ Afternoon meal
- ☐ Evening meal

☐ _____ (fill-in when you did exercise,
☐ _____ example, standing in line, etc)
☐ _____

Day 6 (_____ **)** *write day*

Assessments: *(circle what applies)*
*Surge Posture: 75% or more of the day / 50% of the day / less than 25% of the day
*Core Posture: 75% or more of the day / 50% of the day / less than 25% of the day
Set Posture: 75% or more of the day / 50% of the day / less than 25% of the day
Breathe Posture: 75% or more of the day / 50% of the day / less than 25% of the day

- ☐ Morning meal
- ☐ Afternoon meal
- ☐ Evening meal

☐ _____ (fill-in when you did exercise,
☐ _____ example, standing in line, etc)
☐ _____

Day 7 (_____ **)** *write day*

Assessments: *(circle what applies)*
*Surge Posture: 75% or more of the day / 50% of the day / less than 25% of the day
*Core Posture: 75% or more of the day / 50% of the day / less than 25% of the day
Set Posture: 75% or more of the day / 50% of the day / less than 25% of the day
Breathe Posture: 75% or more of the day / 50% of the day / less than 25% of the day

- ☐ Morning meal
- ☐ Afternoon meal
- ☐ Evening meal

☐ _____ (fill-in when you did exercise,
☐ _____ example, standing in line, etc)
☐ _____

213

Ishio Method ™ Abdominal Rehab (check-off sheet)

Week 3 (/   /20   thru   /   /20   )

Write in your own personal dates.

Seated Pull-ins ™

Rep: 7 reps per set. Breathe in, (allowing your abs to relax), then as you breathe out, pull-in your abs as far in as possible)

Day 1 (_____ **)** *write day*

> **Important:** Wear your Sillo Belly Wrap ™ every night, (crossing in the front).

Assessments: *(circle what applies)*
*Surge Posture: 75% or more of the day / 50% of the day / less than 25% of the day
*Core Posture: 75% or more of the day / 50% of the day / less than 25% of the day
Set Posture: 75% or more of the day / 50% of the day / less than 25% of the day
Breathe Posture: 75% or more of the day / 50% of the day / less than 25% of the day

☐ Morning meal
☐ Afternoon meal
☐ Evening meal

☐ _____ (fill-in when you did exercise,
☐ _____ example, standing in line, etc)
☐ _____

Day 2 (_____ **)** *write day*

Assessments: *(circle what applies)*
*Surge Posture: 75% or more of the day / 50% of the day / less than 25% of the day
*Core Posture: 75% or more of the day / 50% of the day / less than 25% of the day
Set Posture: 75% or more of the day / 50% of the day / less than 25% of the day
Breathe Posture: 75% or more of the day / 50% of the day / less than 25% of the day

☐ Morning meal
☐ Afternoon meal
☐ Evening meal

☐ _____ (fill-in when you did exercise,
☐ _____ example, standing in line, etc)
☐ _____

Day 3 (_____ **)** *write day*

Assessments: *(circle what applies)*
*Surge Posture: 75% or more of the day / 50% of the day / less than 25% of the day
*Core Posture: 75% or more of the day / 50% of the day / less than 25% of the day
Set Posture: 75% or more of the day / 50% of the day / less than 25% of the day
Breathe Posture: 75% or more of the day / 50% of the day / less than 25% of the day

☐ Morning meal
☐ Afternoon meal
☐ Evening meal

☐ _____ (fill-in when you did exercise,
☐ _____ example, standing in line, etc)
☐ _____

Day 4 (_____ **)** *write day*

Assessments: *(circle what applies)*
*Surge Posture: 75% or more of the day / 50% of the day / less than 25% of the day
*Core Posture: 75% or more of the day / 50% of the day / less than 25% of the day
Set Posture: 75% or more of the day / 50% of the day / less than 25% of the day
Breathe Posture: 75% or more of the day / 50% of the day / less than 25% of the day

☐ Morning meal
☐ Afternoon meal
☐ Evening meal

☐ _____ (fill-in when you did exercise,
☐ _____ example, standing in line, etc)
☐ _____

Ishio Method ™ Abdominal Rehab (check-off sheet)

Week 3 (/   /20   thru   /   /20   )

Write in your own personal dates.

Seated Pull-ins ™

Rep: 7 reps per set. Breathe in, (allowing your abs to relax), then as you breathe out, pull-in your abs as far in as possible)

Day 5 (_____ **)** *write day*

> **Important:** Wear your Sillo Belly Wrap ™ every night, (crossing in the front).

Assessments: *(circle what applies)*
*Surge Posture: 75% or more of the day / 50% of the day / less than 25% of the day
*Core Posture: 75% or more of the day / 50% of the day / less than 25% of the day
Set Posture: 75% or more of the day / 50% of the day / less than 25% of the day
Breathe Posture: 75% or more of the day / 50% of the day / less than 25% of the day

☐ Morning meal
☐ Afternoon meal
☐ Evening meal

☐ _____ (fill-in when you did exercise,
☐ _____ example, standing in line, etc)
☐ _____

Day 6 (_____ **)** *write day*

Assessments: *(circle what applies)*
*Surge Posture: 75% or more of the day / 50% of the day / less than 25% of the day
*Core Posture: 75% or more of the day / 50% of the day / less than 25% of the day
Set Posture: 75% or more of the day / 50% of the day / less than 25% of the day
Breathe Posture: 75% or more of the day / 50% of the day / less than 25% of the day

☐ Morning meal
☐ Afternoon meal
☐ Evening meal

☐ _____ (fill-in when you did exercise,
☐ _____ example, standing in line, etc)
☐ _____

Day 7 (_____ **)** *write day*

Assessments: *(circle what applies)*
*Surge Posture: 75% or more of the day / 50% of the day / less than 25% of the day
*Core Posture: 75% or more of the day / 50% of the day / less than 25% of the day
Set Posture: 75% or more of the day / 50% of the day / less than 25% of the day
Breathe Posture: 75% or more of the day / 50% of the day / less than 25% of the day

☐ Morning meal
☐ Afternoon meal
☐ Evening meal

☐ _____ (fill-in when you did exercise,
☐ _____ example, standing in line, etc)
☐ _____

Ishio Method ™ Abdominal Rehab (check-off sheet)

Week 4 (__/__ /20 thru __/__ /20)

Write in your own personal dates.

Seated Pull-ins ™

Rep: 7 reps per set. Breathe in, (allowing your abs to relax), then as you breathe out, pull-in your abs as far in as possible)

Day 1 (_____ **)** *write day*

> **Important:** Wear your Sillo Belly Wrap ™ every night, (crossing in the front).

Assessments: *(circle what applies)*
*Surge Posture: 75% or more of the day / 50% of the day / less than 25% of the day
*Core Posture: 75% or more of the day / 50% of the day / less than 25% of the day
Set Posture: 75% or more of the day / 50% of the day / less than 25% of the day
Breathe Posture: 75% or more of the day / 50% of the day / less than 25% of the day

☐ Morning meal
☐ Afternoon meal
☐ Evening meal

☐ _____
☐ _____
☐ _____

(fill-in when you did exercise, example, standing in line, etc)

Day 2 (_____ **)** *write day*

Assessments: *(circle what applies)*
*Surge Posture: 75% or more of the day / 50% of the day / less than 25% of the day
*Core Posture: 75% or more of the day / 50% of the day / less than 25% of the day
Set Posture: 75% or more of the day / 50% of the day / less than 25% of the day
Breathe Posture: 75% or more of the day / 50% of the day / less than 25% of the day

☐ Morning meal
☐ Afternoon meal
☐ Evening meal

☐ _____
☐ _____
☐ _____

(fill-in when you did exercise, example, standing in line, etc)

Day 3 (_____ **)** *write day*

Assessments: *(circle what applies)*
*Surge Posture: 75% or more of the day / 50% of the day / less than 25% of the day
*Core Posture: 75% or more of the day / 50% of the day / less than 25% of the day
Set Posture: 75% or more of the day / 50% of the day / less than 25% of the day
Breathe Posture: 75% or more of the day / 50% of the day / less than 25% of the day

☐ Morning meal
☐ Afternoon meal
☐ Evening meal

☐ _____
☐ _____
☐ _____

(fill-in when you did exercise, example, standing in line, etc)

Day 4 (_____ **)** *write day*

Assessments: *(circle what applies)*
*Surge Posture: 75% or more of the day / 50% of the day / less than 25% of the day
*Core Posture: 75% or more of the day / 50% of the day / less than 25% of the day
Set Posture: 75% or more of the day / 50% of the day / less than 25% of the day
Breathe Posture: 75% or more of the day / 50% of the day / less than 25% of the day

☐ Morning meal
☐ Afternoon meal
☐ Evening meal

☐ _____
☐ _____
☐ _____

(fill-in when you did exercise, example, standing in line, etc)

216

Ishio Method ™ Abdominal Rehab (check-off sheet)

Week 4 (/ /20 thru / /20)

Write in your own personal dates.

Seated Pull-ins ™

Rep: 7 reps per set. Breathe in, (allowing your abs to relax), then as you breathe out, pull-in your abs as far in as possible)

Day 5 ( ) *write day*

Important: Wear your Sillo Belly Wrap ™ every night, (crossing in the front).

Assessments: *(circle what applies)*
*Surge Posture: 75% or more of the day / 50% of the day / less than 25% of the day
*Core Posture: 75% or more of the day / 50% of the day / less than 25% of the day
Set Posture: 75% or more of the day / 50% of the day / less than 25% of the day
Breathe Posture: 75% or more of the day / 50% of the day / less than 25% of the day

☐ Morning meal
☐ Afternoon meal
☐ Evening meal

☐ _____ (fill-in when you did exercise,
☐ _____ example, standing in line, etc)
☐ _____

Day 6 ( ) *write day*

Assessments: *(circle what applies)*
*Surge Posture: 75% or more of the day / 50% of the day / less than 25% of the day
*Core Posture: 75% or more of the day / 50% of the day / less than 25% of the day
Set Posture: 75% or more of the day / 50% of the day / less than 25% of the day
Breathe Posture: 75% or more of the day / 50% of the day / less than 25% of the day

☐ Morning meal
☐ Afternoon meal
☐ Evening meal

☐ _____ (fill-in when you did exercise,
☐ _____ example, standing in line, etc)
☐ _____

Day 7 ( ) *write day*

Assessments: *(circle what applies)*
*Surge Posture: 75% or more of the day / 50% of the day / less than 25% of the day
*Core Posture: 75% or more of the day / 50% of the day / less than 25% of the day
Set Posture: 75% or more of the day / 50% of the day / less than 25% of the day
Breathe Posture: 75% or more of the day / 50% of the day / less than 25% of the day

☐ Morning meal
☐ Afternoon meal
☐ Evening meal

☐ _____ (fill-in when you did exercise,
☐ _____ example, standing in line, etc)
☐ _____

217

Ishio Method ™ Abdominal Rehab (check-off sheet)

Week 5 (/   /20   thru   /   /20   )

Write in your own personal dates.

Adding: Incline Planks ™

Set: 3 sets of 45 seconds each.

Day 1 ( ) *write day*

| **Important:** Wear your Sillo Belly Wrap ™ every night, (crossing in the front). |

Assessments: *(circle what applies)*
*Surge Posture: 75% or more of the day / 50% of the day / less than 25% of the day
*Core Posture: 75% or more of the day / 50% of the day / less than 25% of the day
Set Posture: 75% or more of the day / 50% of the day / less than 25% of the day
Breathe Posture: 75% or more of the day / 50% of the day / less than 25% of the day

Seated Pull-ins ™ - How many times today _____.
Incline Planks ™ - How many sets today _____, how many seconds each set _____.

Day 2 ( ) *write day*

Assessments: *(circle what applies)*
*Surge Posture: 75% or more of the day / 50% of the day / less than 25% of the day
*Core Posture: 75% or more of the day / 50% of the day / less than 25% of the day
Set Posture: 75% or more of the day / 50% of the day / less than 25% of the day
Breathe Posture: 75% or more of the day / 50% of the day / less than 25% of the day

Seated Pull-ins ™ - How many times today _____.
Incline Planks ™ - How many sets today _____, how many seconds each set _____.

Day 3 ( ) *write day*

Assessments: *(circle what applies)*
*Surge Posture: 75% or more of the day / 50% of the day / less than 25% of the day
*Core Posture: 75% or more of the day / 50% of the day / less than 25% of the day
Set Posture: 75% or more of the day / 50% of the day / less than 25% of the day
Breathe Posture: 75% or more of the day / 50% of the day / less than 25% of the day

Seated Pull-ins ™ - How many times today _____.
Incline Planks ™ - How many sets today _____, how many seconds each set _____.

Day 4 ( ) *write day*

Assessments: *(circle what applies)*
*Surge Posture: 75% or more of the day / 50% of the day / less than 25% of the day
*Core Posture: 75% or more of the day / 50% of the day / less than 25% of the day
Set Posture: 75% or more of the day / 50% of the day / less than 25% of the day
Breathe Posture: 75% or more of the day / 50% of the day / less than 25% of the day

Seated Pull-ins ™ - How many times today _____.
Incline Planks ™ - How many sets today _____, how many seconds each set _____.

Ishio Method ™ Abdominal Rehab (check-off sheet)

Week 5 (/ /20 thru / /20)

Write in your own personal dates.

Adding: Incline Planks ™

Set: 3 sets of 45 seconds each.

Day 5 (**)** *write day*

| **Important:** Wear your Sillo Belly Wrap ™ every night, (crossing in the front). |

Assessments: *(circle what applies)*
*Surge Posture: 75% or more of the day / 50% of the day / less than 25% of the day
*Core Posture: 75% or more of the day / 50% of the day / less than 25% of the day
Set Posture: 75% or more of the day / 50% of the day / less than 25% of the day
Breathe Posture: 75% or more of the day / 50% of the day / less than 25% of the day

Seated Pull-ins ™ - How many times today _____.
Incline Planks ™ - How many sets today _____, how many seconds each set _____.

Day 6 (**)** *write day*

Assessments: *(circle what applies)*
*Surge Posture: 75% or more of the day / 50% of the day / less than 25% of the day
*Core Posture: 75% or more of the day / 50% of the day / less than 25% of the day
Set Posture: 75% or more of the day / 50% of the day / less than 25% of the day
Breathe Posture: 75% or more of the day / 50% of the day / less than 25% of the day

Seated Pull-ins ™ - How many times today _____.
Incline Planks ™ - How many sets today _____, how many seconds each set _____.

Day 7 (**)** *write day*

Assessments: *(circle what applies)*
*Surge Posture: 75% or more of the day / 50% of the day / less than 25% of the day
*Core Posture: 75% or more of the day / 50% of the day / less than 25% of the day
Set Posture: 75% or more of the day / 50% of the day / less than 25% of the day
Breathe Posture: 75% or more of the day / 50% of the day / less than 25% of the day

Seated Pull-ins ™ - How many times today _____.
Incline Planks ™ - How many sets today _____, how many seconds each set _____.

219

Ishio Method ™ Abdominal Rehab (check-off sheet)

Week 6 (/ /20 thru / /20)

Write in your own personal dates.

Adding: Incline Planks ™

Set: 3 sets of 45 seconds each.

Day 1 (**)** *write day*

| **Important:** Wear your Sillo Belly Wrap ™ every night, (crossing in the front). |

Assessments: *(circle what applies)*
*Surge Posture: 75% or more of the day / 50% of the day / less than 25% of the day
*Core Posture: 75% or more of the day / 50% of the day / less than 25% of the day
Set Posture: 75% or more of the day / 50% of the day / less than 25% of the day
Breathe Posture: 75% or more of the day / 50% of the day / less than 25% of the day

Seated Pull-ins ™ - How many times today _____.
Incline Planks ™ - How many sets today _____, how many seconds each set _____.

Day 2 (**)** *write day*

Assessments: *(circle what applies)*
*Surge Posture: 75% or more of the day / 50% of the day / less than 25% of the day
*Core Posture: 75% or more of the day / 50% of the day / less than 25% of the day
Set Posture: 75% or more of the day / 50% of the day / less than 25% of the day
Breathe Posture: 75% or more of the day / 50% of the day / less than 25% of the day

Seated Pull-ins ™ - How many times today _____.
Incline Planks ™ - How many sets today _____, how many seconds each set _____.

Day 3 (**)** *write day*

Assessments: *(circle what applies)*
*Surge Posture: 75% or more of the day / 50% of the day / less than 25% of the day
*Core Posture: 75% or more of the day / 50% of the day / less than 25% of the day
Set Posture: 75% or more of the day / 50% of the day / less than 25% of the day
Breathe Posture: 75% or more of the day / 50% of the day / less than 25% of the day

Seated Pull-ins ™ - How many times today _____.
Incline Planks ™ - How many sets today _____, how many seconds each set _____.

Day 4 (**)** *write day*

Assessments: *(circle what applies)*
*Surge Posture: 75% or more of the day / 50% of the day / less than 25% of the day
*Core Posture: 75% or more of the day / 50% of the day / less than 25% of the day
Set Posture: 75% or more of the day / 50% of the day / less than 25% of the day
Breathe Posture: 75% or more of the day / 50% of the day / less than 25% of the day

Seated Pull-ins ™ - How many times today _____.
Incline Planks ™ - How many sets today _____, how many seconds each set _____.

Ishio Method ™ Abdominal Rehab (check-off sheet)

Week 6 (/ /20 thru / /20)

Write in your own personal dates.

Adding: Incline Planks ™

Set: 3 sets of 45 seconds each.

Day 5 ( ) *write day*

| **Important:** Wear your Sillo Belly Wrap ™ every night, (crossing in the front). |

Assessments: *(circle what applies)*
*Surge Posture: 75% or more of the day / 50% of the day / less than 25% of the day
*Core Posture: 75% or more of the day / 50% of the day / less than 25% of the day
Set Posture: 75% or more of the day / 50% of the day / less than 25% of the day
Breathe Posture: 75% or more of the day / 50% of the day / less than 25% of the day

Seated Pull-ins ™ - How many times today _____.
Incline Planks ™ - How many sets today _____, how many seconds each set _____.

Day 6 ( ) *write day*

Assessments: *(circle what applies)*
*Surge Posture: 75% or more of the day / 50% of the day / less than 25% of the day
*Core Posture: 75% or more of the day / 50% of the day / less than 25% of the day
Set Posture: 75% or more of the day / 50% of the day / less than 25% of the day
Breathe Posture: 75% or more of the day / 50% of the day / less than 25% of the day

Seated Pull-ins ™ - How many times today _____.
Incline Planks ™ - How many sets today _____, how many seconds each set _____.

Day 7 ( ) *write day*

Assessments: *(circle what applies)*
*Surge Posture: 75% or more of the day / 50% of the day / less than 25% of the day
*Core Posture: 75% or more of the day / 50% of the day / less than 25% of the day
Set Posture: 75% or more of the day / 50% of the day / less than 25% of the day
Breathe Posture: 75% or more of the day / 50% of the day / less than 25% of the day

Seated Pull-ins ™ - How many times today _____.
Incline Planks ™ - How many sets today _____, how many seconds each set _____.

Ishio Method ™ Abdominal Rehab (check-off sheet)

Week 7 (/ /20 thru / /20)

Write in your own personal dates.

Adding: Incline Planks ™

Set: 3 sets of 45 seconds each.

Day 1 ( ) *write day*

> **Important:** Wear your Sillo Belly Wrap ™ every night, (crossing in the front).

Assessments: *(circle what applies)*
*Surge Posture: 75% or more of the day / 50% of the day / less than 25% of the day
*Core Posture: 75% or more of the day / 50% of the day / less than 25% of the day
Set Posture: 75% or more of the day / 50% of the day / less than 25% of the day
Breathe Posture: 75% or more of the day / 50% of the day / less than 25% of the day

Seated Pull-ins ™ - How many times today _____.
Incline Planks ™ - How many sets today _____, how many seconds each set _____.

Day 2 ( ) *write day*

Assessments: *(circle what applies)*
*Surge Posture: 75% or more of the day / 50% of the day / less than 25% of the day
*Core Posture: 75% or more of the day / 50% of the day / less than 25% of the day
Set Posture: 75% or more of the day / 50% of the day / less than 25% of the day
Breathe Posture: 75% or more of the day / 50% of the day / less than 25% of the day

Seated Pull-ins ™ - How many times today _____.
Incline Planks ™ - How many sets today _____, how many seconds each set _____.

Day 3 ( ) *write day*

Assessments: *(circle what applies)*
*Surge Posture: 75% or more of the day / 50% of the day / less than 25% of the day
*Core Posture: 75% or more of the day / 50% of the day / less than 25% of the day
Set Posture: 75% or more of the day / 50% of the day / less than 25% of the day
Breathe Posture: 75% or more of the day / 50% of the day / less than 25% of the day

Seated Pull-ins ™ - How many times today _____.
Incline Planks ™ - How many sets today _____, how many seconds each set _____.

Day 4 ( ) *write day*

Assessments: *(circle what applies)*
*Surge Posture: 75% or more of the day / 50% of the day / less than 25% of the day
*Core Posture: 75% or more of the day / 50% of the day / less than 25% of the day
Set Posture: 75% or more of the day / 50% of the day / less than 25% of the day
Breathe Posture: 75% or more of the day / 50% of the day / less than 25% of the day

Seated Pull-ins ™ - How many times today _____.
Incline Planks ™ - How many sets today _____, how many seconds each set _____.

Ishio Method ™ Abdominal Rehab (check-off sheet)

Week 7 (/   /20   thru   /   /20   )

Write in your own personal dates.

Adding: Incline Planks ™

Set: 3 sets of 45 seconds each.

Day 5 (   ) *write day*

Important: Wear your Sillo Belly Wrap ™ every night, (crossing in the front).

Assessments: *(circle what applies)*
*Surge Posture: 75% or more of the day / 50% of the day / less than 25% of the day
*Core Posture: 75% or more of the day / 50% of the day / less than 25% of the day
Set Posture: 75% or more of the day / 50% of the day / less than 25% of the day
Breathe Posture: 75% or more of the day / 50% of the day / less than 25% of the day

Seated Pull-ins ™ - How many times today _____.
Incline Planks ™ - How many sets today _____, how many seconds each set _____.

Day 6 (   ) *write day*

Assessments: *(circle what applies)*
*Surge Posture: 75% or more of the day / 50% of the day / less than 25% of the day
*Core Posture: 75% or more of the day / 50% of the day / less than 25% of the day
Set Posture: 75% or more of the day / 50% of the day / less than 25% of the day
Breathe Posture: 75% or more of the day / 50% of the day / less than 25% of the day

Seated Pull-ins ™ - How many times today _____.
Incline Planks ™ - How many sets today _____, how many seconds each set _____.

Day 7 (   ) *write day*

Assessments: *(circle what applies)*
*Surge Posture: 75% or more of the day / 50% of the day / less than 25% of the day
*Core Posture: 75% or more of the day / 50% of the day / less than 25% of the day
Set Posture: 75% or more of the day / 50% of the day / less than 25% of the day
Breathe Posture: 75% or more of the day / 50% of the day / less than 25% of the day

Seated Pull-ins ™ - How many times today _____.
Incline Planks ™ - How many sets today _____, how many seconds each set _____.

223

Ishio Method ™ Abdominal Rehab (check-off sheet)

Week 8 (/   /20   thru   /   /20   )

Write in your own personal dates.

Adding: Incline Planks ™

Set: 3 sets of 45 seconds each.

Day 1 (_____ **)** *write day*

> **Important:** Wear your Sillo Belly Wrap ™ every night, (crossing in the front).

Assessments: *(circle what applies)*
*Surge Posture: 75% or more of the day / 50% of the day / less than 25% of the day
*Core Posture: 75% or more of the day / 50% of the day / less than 25% of the day
Set Posture: 75% or more of the day / 50% of the day / less than 25% of the day
Breathe Posture: 75% or more of the day / 50% of the day / less than 25% of the day

Seated Pull-ins ™ - How many times today _____.
Incline Planks ™ - How many sets today _____, how many seconds each set _____.

Day 2 (_____ **)** *write day*

Assessments: *(circle what applies)*
*Surge Posture: 75% or more of the day / 50% of the day / less than 25% of the day
*Core Posture: 75% or more of the day / 50% of the day / less than 25% of the day
Set Posture: 75% or more of the day / 50% of the day / less than 25% of the day
Breathe Posture: 75% or more of the day / 50% of the day / less than 25% of the day

Seated Pull-ins ™ - How many times today _____.
Incline Planks ™ - How many sets today _____, how many seconds each set _____.

Day 3 (_____ **)** *write day*

Assessments: *(circle what applies)*
*Surge Posture: 75% or more of the day / 50% of the day / less than 25% of the day
*Core Posture: 75% or more of the day / 50% of the day / less than 25% of the day
Set Posture: 75% or more of the day / 50% of the day / less than 25% of the day
Breathe Posture: 75% or more of the day / 50% of the day / less than 25% of the day

Seated Pull-ins ™ - How many times today _____.
Incline Planks ™ - How many sets today _____, how many seconds each set _____.

Day 4 (_____ **)** *write day*

Assessments: *(circle what applies)*
*Surge Posture: 75% or more of the day / 50% of the day / less than 25% of the day
*Core Posture: 75% or more of the day / 50% of the day / less than 25% of the day
Set Posture: 75% or more of the day / 50% of the day / less than 25% of the day
Breathe Posture: 75% or more of the day / 50% of the day / less than 25% of the day

Seated Pull-ins ™ - How many times today _____.
Incline Planks ™ - How many sets today _____, how many seconds each set _____.

Ishio Method ™ Abdominal Rehab (check-off sheet)

Week 8 (/ /20 thru / /20)

Write in your own personal dates.

Adding: Incline Planks ™

Set: 3 sets of 45 seconds each.

Day 5 (_____ **)** *write day*

| **Important:** Wear your Sillo Belly Wrap ™ every night, (crossing in the front). |

Assessments: *(circle what applies)*
*Surge Posture: 75% or more of the day / 50% of the day / less than 25% of the day
*Core Posture: 75% or more of the day / 50% of the day / less than 25% of the day
Set Posture: 75% or more of the day / 50% of the day / less than 25% of the day
Breathe Posture: 75% or more of the day / 50% of the day / less than 25% of the day

Seated Pull-ins ™ - How many times today _____.
Incline Planks ™ - How many sets today _____, how many seconds each set _____.

Day 6 (_____ **)** *write day*

Assessments: *(circle what applies)*
*Surge Posture: 75% or more of the day / 50% of the day / less than 25% of the day
*Core Posture: 75% or more of the day / 50% of the day / less than 25% of the day
Set Posture: 75% or more of the day / 50% of the day / less than 25% of the day
Breathe Posture: 75% or more of the day / 50% of the day / less than 25% of the day

Seated Pull-ins ™ - How many times today _____.
Incline Planks ™ - How many sets today _____, how many seconds each set _____.

Day 7 (_____ **)** *write day*

Assessments: *(circle what applies)*
*Surge Posture: 75% or more of the day / 50% of the day / less than 25% of the day
*Core Posture: 75% or more of the day / 50% of the day / less than 25% of the day
Set Posture: 75% or more of the day / 50% of the day / less than 25% of the day
Breathe Posture: 75% or more of the day / 50% of the day / less than 25% of the day

Seated Pull-ins ™ - How many times today _____.
Incline Planks ™ - How many sets today _____, how many seconds each set _____.

Ishio Method ™ Abdominal Rehab (check-off sheet)

Week 9 (/   /20   thru   /   /20   )

Write in your own personal dates.

Standing Tilts ™ and Half and Half Planks ™

Set: Standing Tilts ™ - 10 pulse repetitions / Half and Half Planks ™ - 3 sets of 20 seconds (each side)

Day 1 (_____) *write day*

> **Important:** Wear your Sillo Belly Wrap ™ every night, (crossing in the front).

Assessments: *(circle what applies)*
*Surge Posture: 75% or more of the day / 50% of the day / less than 25% of the day
*Core Posture: 75% or more of the day / 50% of the day / less than 25% of the day
Set Posture: 75% or more of the day / 50% of the day / less than 25% of the day
Breathe Posture: 75% or more of the day / 50% of the day / less than 25% of the day

Standing Tilts ™ - How many sets today_____.
Half and Half Planks ™ - How many sets today_____, how many seconds each set _____.

Day 2 (_____) *write day*

Assessments: *(circle what applies)*
*Surge Posture: 75% or more of the day / 50% of the day / less than 25% of the day
*Core Posture: 75% or more of the day / 50% of the day / less than 25% of the day
Set Posture: 75% or more of the day / 50% of the day / less than 25% of the day
Breathe Posture: 75% or more of the day / 50% of the day / less than 25% of the day

Standing Tilts ™ - How many sets today_____.
Half and Half Planks ™ - How many sets today_____, how many seconds each set _____.

Day 3 (_____) *write day*

Assessments: *(circle what applies)*
*Surge Posture: 75% or more of the day / 50% of the day / less than 25% of the day
*Core Posture: 75% or more of the day / 50% of the day / less than 25% of the day
Set Posture: 75% or more of the day / 50% of the day / less than 25% of the day
Breathe Posture: 75% or more of the day / 50% of the day / less than 25% of the day

Standing Tilts ™ - How many sets today_____.
Half and Half Planks ™ - How many sets today_____, how many seconds each set _____.

Day 4 (_____) *write day*

Assessments: *(circle what applies)*
*Surge Posture: 75% or more of the day / 50% of the day / less than 25% of the day
*Core Posture: 75% or more of the day / 50% of the day / less than 25% of the day
Set Posture: 75% or more of the day / 50% of the day / less than 25% of the day
Breathe Posture: 75% or more of the day / 50% of the day / less than 25% of the day

Standing Tilts ™ - How many sets today_____.
Half and Half Planks ™ - How many sets today_____, how many seconds each set _____.

226

Ishio Method ™ Abdominal Rehab (check-off sheet)

Week 9 (/   /20   thru   /   /20   )
Write in your own personal dates.

Standing Tilts ™ and Half and Half Planks ™

Set: Standing Tilts ™ - 10 pulse repetitions / Half and Half Planks ™ - 3 sets of 20 seconds (each side)

Day 5 (_____ **)** *write day*

| **Important:** Wear your Sillo Belly Wrap ™ every night, (crossing in the front). |

Assessments: *(circle what applies)*
*Surge Posture: 75% or more of the day / 50% of the day / less than 25% of the day
*Core Posture: 75% or more of the day / 50% of the day / less than 25% of the day
Set Posture: 75% or more of the day / 50% of the day / less than 25% of the day
Breathe Posture: 75% or more of the day / 50% of the day / less than 25% of the day

Standing Tilts ™ - How many sets today_____.
Half and Half Planks ™ - How many sets today_____, how many seconds each set _____.

Day 6 (_____ **)** *write day*

Assessments: *(circle what applies)*
*Surge Posture: 75% or more of the day / 50% of the day / less than 25% of the day
*Core Posture: 75% or more of the day / 50% of the day / less than 25% of the day
Set Posture: 75% or more of the day / 50% of the day / less than 25% of the day
Breathe Posture: 75% or more of the day / 50% of the day / less than 25% of the day

Standing Tilts ™ - How many sets today_____.
Half and Half Planks ™ - How many sets today_____, how many seconds each set _____.

Day 7 (_____ **)** *write day*

Assessments: *(circle what applies)*
*Surge Posture: 75% or more of the day / 50% of the day / less than 25% of the day
*Core Posture: 75% or more of the day / 50% of the day / less than 25% of the day
Set Posture: 75% or more of the day / 50% of the day / less than 25% of the day
Breathe Posture: 75% or more of the day / 50% of the day / less than 25% of the day

Standing Tilts ™ - How many sets today_____.
Half and Half Planks ™ - How many sets today_____, how many seconds each set _____.

Ishio Method ™ Abdominal Rehab (check-off sheet)

Week 10 (/   /20   thru   /   /20   )   *Write in your own personal dates.*

Standing Tilts ™ and Half and Half Planks ™

Set: Standing Tilts ™ - 10 pulse repetitions / Half and Half Planks ™ - 3 sets of 20 seconds (each side)

Day 1 ( ) *write day*

Important: Wear your Sillo Belly Wrap ™ every night, (crossing in the front).

Assessments: *(circle what applies)*
*Surge Posture: 75% or more of the day / 50% of the day / less than 25% of the day
*Core Posture: 75% or more of the day / 50% of the day / less than 25% of the day
Set Posture: 75% or more of the day / 50% of the day / less than 25% of the day
Breathe Posture: 75% or more of the day / 50% of the day / less than 25% of the day

Standing Tilts ™ - How many sets today_____.
Half and Half Planks ™ - How many sets today_____, how many seconds each set _____.

Day 2 ( ) *write day*

Assessments: *(circle what applies)*
*Surge Posture: 75% or more of the day / 50% of the day / less than 25% of the day
*Core Posture: 75% or more of the day / 50% of the day / less than 25% of the day
Set Posture: 75% or more of the day / 50% of the day / less than 25% of the day
Breathe Posture: 75% or more of the day / 50% of the day / less than 25% of the day

Standing Tilts ™ - How many sets today_____.
Half and Half Planks ™ - How many sets today_____, how many seconds each set _____.

Day 3 ( ) *write day*

Assessments: *(circle what applies)*
*Surge Posture: 75% or more of the day / 50% of the day / less than 25% of the day
*Core Posture: 75% or more of the day / 50% of the day / less than 25% of the day
Set Posture: 75% or more of the day / 50% of the day / less than 25% of the day
Breathe Posture: 75% or more of the day / 50% of the day / less than 25% of the day

Standing Tilts ™ - How many sets today_____.
Half and Half Planks ™ - How many sets today_____, how many seconds each set _____.

Day 4 ( ) *write day*

Assessments: *(circle what applies)*
*Surge Posture: 75% or more of the day / 50% of the day / less than 25% of the day
*Core Posture: 75% or more of the day / 50% of the day / less than 25% of the day
Set Posture: 75% or more of the day / 50% of the day / less than 25% of the day
Breathe Posture: 75% or more of the day / 50% of the day / less than 25% of the day

Standing Tilts ™ - How many sets today_____.
Half and Half Planks ™ - How many sets today_____, how many seconds each set _____.

Ishio Method ™ Abdominal Rehab (check-off sheet)

Week 10 (/   /20   thru   /   /20   )

Write in your own personal dates.

Standing Tilts ™ and Half and Half Planks ™

Set: Standing Tilts ™ - 10 pulse repetitions / Half and Half Planks ™ - 3 sets of 20 seconds (each side)

Day 5 (**)** *write day*

Important: Wear your Sillo Belly Wrap ™ every night, (crossing in the front).

Assessments: *(circle what applies)*
*Surge Posture: 75% or more of the day / 50% of the day / less than 25% of the day
*Core Posture: 75% or more of the day / 50% of the day / less than 25% of the day
Set Posture: 75% or more of the day / 50% of the day / less than 25% of the day
Breathe Posture: 75% or more of the day / 50% of the day / less than 25% of the day

Standing Tilts ™ - How many sets today_____.
Half and Half Planks ™ - How many sets today_____, how many seconds each set _____.

Day 6 (**)** *write day*

Assessments: *(circle what applies)*
*Surge Posture: 75% or more of the day / 50% of the day / less than 25% of the day
*Core Posture: 75% or more of the day / 50% of the day / less than 25% of the day
Set Posture: 75% or more of the day / 50% of the day / less than 25% of the day
Breathe Posture: 75% or more of the day / 50% of the day / less than 25% of the day

Standing Tilts ™ - How many sets today_____.
Half and Half Planks ™ - How many sets today_____, how many seconds each set _____.

Day 7 (**)** *write day*

Assessments: *(circle what applies)*
*Surge Posture: 75% or more of the day / 50% of the day / less than 25% of the day
*Core Posture: 75% or more of the day / 50% of the day / less than 25% of the day
Set Posture: 75% or more of the day / 50% of the day / less than 25% of the day
Breathe Posture: 75% or more of the day / 50% of the day / less than 25% of the day

Standing Tilts ™ - How many sets today_____.
Half and Half Planks ™ - How many sets today_____, how many seconds each set _____.

229

Ishio Method ™ Abdominal Rehab (check-off sheet)

Week 11 (/   /20   thru   /   /20   )

Write in your own personal dates.

Standing Tilts ™ and Half and Half Planks ™

Set: Standing Tilts ™ - 10 pulse repetitions / Half and Half Planks ™ - 3 sets of 20 seconds (each side)

Day 1 ( ) *write day*

| **Important:** Wear your Sillo Belly Wrap ™ every night, (crossing in the front). |

Assessments: *(circle what applies)*
*Surge Posture: 75% or more of the day / 50% of the day / less than 25% of the day
*Core Posture: 75% or more of the day / 50% of the day / less than 25% of the day
Set Posture: 75% or more of the day / 50% of the day / less than 25% of the day
Breathe Posture: 75% or more of the day / 50% of the day / less than 25% of the day

Standing Tilts ™ - How many sets today_____.
Half and Half Planks ™ - How many sets today_____, how many seconds each set _____.

Day 2 ( ) *write day*

Assessments: *(circle what applies)*
*Surge Posture: 75% or more of the day / 50% of the day / less than 25% of the day
*Core Posture: 75% or more of the day / 50% of the day / less than 25% of the day
Set Posture: 75% or more of the day / 50% of the day / less than 25% of the day
Breathe Posture: 75% or more of the day / 50% of the day / less than 25% of the day

Standing Tilts ™ - How many sets today_____.
Half and Half Planks ™ - How many sets today_____, how many seconds each set _____.

Day 3 ( ) *write day*

Assessments: *(circle what applies)*
*Surge Posture: 75% or more of the day / 50% of the day / less than 25% of the day
*Core Posture: 75% or more of the day / 50% of the day / less than 25% of the day
Set Posture: 75% or more of the day / 50% of the day / less than 25% of the day
Breathe Posture: 75% or more of the day / 50% of the day / less than 25% of the day

Standing Tilts ™ - How many sets today_____.
Half and Half Planks ™ - How many sets today_____, how many seconds each set _____.

Day 4 ( ) *write day*

Assessments: *(circle what applies)*
*Surge Posture: 75% or more of the day / 50% of the day / less than 25% of the day
*Core Posture: 75% or more of the day / 50% of the day / less than 25% of the day
Set Posture: 75% or more of the day / 50% of the day / less than 25% of the day
Breathe Posture: 75% or more of the day / 50% of the day / less than 25% of the day

Standing Tilts ™ - How many sets today_____.
Half and Half Planks ™ - How many sets today_____, how many seconds each set _____.

Ishio Method ™ Abdominal Rehab (check-off sheet)

Week 11 (/   /20   thru   /   /20   )

Write in your own personal dates.

Standing Tilts ™ and Half and Half Planks ™

Set: Standing Tilts ™ - 10 pulse repetitions / Half and Half Planks ™ - 3 sets of 20 seconds (each side)

Day 5 ( ) *write day*

> **Important:** Wear your Sillo Belly Wrap ™ every night, (crossing in the front).

Assessments: *(circle what applies)*
*Surge Posture: 75% or more of the day / 50% of the day / less than 25% of the day
*Core Posture: 75% or more of the day / 50% of the day / less than 25% of the day
Set Posture: 75% or more of the day / 50% of the day / less than 25% of the day
Breathe Posture: 75% or more of the day / 50% of the day / less than 25% of the day

Standing Tilts ™ - How many sets today_____.
Half and Half Planks ™ - How many sets today_____, how many seconds each set _____.

Day 6 ( ) *write day*

Assessments: *(circle what applies)*
*Surge Posture: 75% or more of the day / 50% of the day / less than 25% of the day
*Core Posture: 75% or more of the day / 50% of the day / less than 25% of the day
Set Posture: 75% or more of the day / 50% of the day / less than 25% of the day
Breathe Posture: 75% or more of the day / 50% of the day / less than 25% of the day

Standing Tilts ™ - How many sets today_____.
Half and Half Planks ™ - How many sets today_____, how many seconds each set _____.

Day 7 ( ) *write day*

Assessments: *(circle what applies)*
*Surge Posture: 75% or more of the day / 50% of the day / less than 25% of the day
*Core Posture: 75% or more of the day / 50% of the day / less than 25% of the day
Set Posture: 75% or more of the day / 50% of the day / less than 25% of the day
Breathe Posture: 75% or more of the day / 50% of the day / less than 25% of the day

Standing Tilts ™ - How many sets today_____.
Half and Half Planks ™ - How many sets today_____, how many seconds each set _____.

Ishio Method ™ Abdominal Rehab (check-off sheet)

Week 12 (__ / __ /20 thru __ / __ /20)

Write in your own personal dates.

Standing Tilts ™ and Half and Half Planks ™

Set: Standing Tilts ™ - 10 pulse repetitions / Half and Half Planks ™ - 3 sets of 20 seconds (each side)

Day 1 (_____ **)** *write day*

> **Important:** Wear your Sillo Belly Wrap ™ every night, (crossing in the front).

Assessments: *(circle what applies)*
*Surge Posture: 75% or more of the day / 50% of the day / less than 25% of the day
*Core Posture: 75% or more of the day / 50% of the day / less than 25% of the day
Set Posture: 75% or more of the day / 50% of the day / less than 25% of the day
Breathe Posture: 75% or more of the day / 50% of the day / less than 25% of the day

Standing Tilts ™ - How many sets today_____.
Half and Half Planks ™ - How many sets today_____, how many seconds each set _____.

Day 2 (_____ **)** *write day*

Assessments: *(circle what applies)*
*Surge Posture: 75% or more of the day / 50% of the day / less than 25% of the day
*Core Posture: 75% or more of the day / 50% of the day / less than 25% of the day
Set Posture: 75% or more of the day / 50% of the day / less than 25% of the day
Breathe Posture: 75% or more of the day / 50% of the day / less than 25% of the day

Standing Tilts ™ - How many sets today_____.
Half and Half Planks ™ - How many sets today_____, how many seconds each set _____.

Day 3 (_____ **)** *write day*

Assessments: *(circle what applies)*
*Surge Posture: 75% or more of the day / 50% of the day / less than 25% of the day
*Core Posture: 75% or more of the day / 50% of the day / less than 25% of the day
Set Posture: 75% or more of the day / 50% of the day / less than 25% of the day
Breathe Posture: 75% or more of the day / 50% of the day / less than 25% of the day

Standing Tilts ™ - How many sets today_____.
Half and Half Planks ™ - How many sets today_____, how many seconds each set _____.

Day 4 (_____ **)** *write day*

Assessments: *(circle what applies)*
*Surge Posture: 75% or more of the day / 50% of the day / less than 25% of the day
*Core Posture: 75% or more of the day / 50% of the day / less than 25% of the day
Set Posture: 75% or more of the day / 50% of the day / less than 25% of the day
Breathe Posture: 75% or more of the day / 50% of the day / less than 25% of the day

Standing Tilts ™ - How many sets today_____.
Half and Half Planks ™ - How many sets today_____, how many seconds each set _____.

Ishio Method ™ Abdominal Rehab (check-off sheet)

Week 12 (/ /20   thru   / /20   )

Write in your own personal dates.

Standing Tilts ™ and Half and Half Planks ™

Set: Standing Tilts ™ - 10 pulse repetitions / Half and Half Planks ™ - 3 sets of 20 seconds (each side)

Day 5 (   ) *write day*

Important: Wear your Sillo Belly Wrap ™ every night, (crossing in the front).

Assessments: *(circle what applies)*
*Surge Posture: 75% or more of the day / 50% of the day / less than 25% of the day
*Core Posture: 75% or more of the day / 50% of the day / less than 25% of the day
Set Posture: 75% or more of the day / 50% of the day / less than 25% of the day
Breathe Posture: 75% or more of the day / 50% of the day / less than 25% of the day

Standing Tilts ™ - How many sets today_____.
Half and Half Planks ™ - How many sets today_____, how many seconds each set _____.

Day 6 (   ) *write day*

Assessments: *(circle what applies)*
*Surge Posture: 75% or more of the day / 50% of the day / less than 25% of the day
*Core Posture: 75% or more of the day / 50% of the day / less than 25% of the day
Set Posture: 75% or more of the day / 50% of the day / less than 25% of the day
Breathe Posture: 75% or more of the day / 50% of the day / less than 25% of the day

Standing Tilts ™ - How many sets today_____.
Half and Half Planks ™ - How many sets today_____, how many seconds each set _____.

Day 7 (   ) *write day*

Assessments: *(circle what applies)*
*Surge Posture: 75% or more of the day / 50% of the day / less than 25% of the day
*Core Posture: 75% or more of the day / 50% of the day / less than 25% of the day
Set Posture: 75% or more of the day / 50% of the day / less than 25% of the day
Breathe Posture: 75% or more of the day / 50% of the day / less than 25% of the day

Standing Tilts ™ - How many sets today_____.
Half and Half Planks ™ - How many sets today_____, how many seconds each set _____.

233

Ishio Method ™ Abdominal Rehab (check-off sheet)

Week 13 (/ /20   thru   / /20   )

Write in your own personal dates.

Standing Tilts ™ and Half and Half Planks ™

Set: Standing Tilts ™ - 10 pulse repetitions / Half and Half Planks ™ - 3 sets of 20 seconds (each side)

Day 1 (_____ **)** *write day*

| **Important:** Wear your Sillo Belly Wrap ™ every night, (**start crossing in the back**). |

Assessments: *(circle what applies)*
*Surge Posture: 75% or more of the day / 50% of the day / less than 25% of the day
*Core Posture: 75% or more of the day / 50% of the day / less than 25% of the day
Set Posture: 75% or more of the day / 50% of the day / less than 25% of the day
Breathe Posture: 75% or more of the day / 50% of the day / less than 25% of the day

Standing Tilts ™ - How many sets today_____.
Half and Half Planks ™ - How many sets today_____, how many seconds each set _____.

Day 2 (_____ **)** *write day*

Assessments: *(circle what applies)*
*Surge Posture: 75% or more of the day / 50% of the day / less than 25% of the day
*Core Posture: 75% or more of the day / 50% of the day / less than 25% of the day
Set Posture: 75% or more of the day / 50% of the day / less than 25% of the day
Breathe Posture: 75% or more of the day / 50% of the day / less than 25% of the day

Standing Tilts ™ - How many sets today_____.
Half and Half Planks ™ - How many sets today_____, how many seconds each set _____.

Day 3 (_____ **)** *write day*

Assessments: *(circle what applies)*
*Surge Posture: 75% or more of the day / 50% of the day / less than 25% of the day
*Core Posture: 75% or more of the day / 50% of the day / less than 25% of the day
Set Posture: 75% or more of the day / 50% of the day / less than 25% of the day
Breathe Posture: 75% or more of the day / 50% of the day / less than 25% of the day

Standing Tilts ™ - How many sets today_____.
Half and Half Planks ™ - How many sets today_____, how many seconds each set _____.

Day 4 (_____ **)** *write day*

Assessments: *(circle what applies)*
*Surge Posture: 75% or more of the day / 50% of the day / less than 25% of the day
*Core Posture: 75% or more of the day / 50% of the day / less than 25% of the day
Set Posture: 75% or more of the day / 50% of the day / less than 25% of the day
Breathe Posture: 75% or more of the day / 50% of the day / less than 25% of the day

Standing Tilts ™ - How many sets today_____.
Half and Half Planks ™ - How many sets today_____, how many seconds each set _____.

234

Ishio Method ™ Abdominal Rehab (check-off sheet)

Week 13 (/ /20 thru / /20)

Write in your own personal dates.

Standing Tilts ™ and Half and Half Planks ™

Set: Standing Tilts ™ - 10 pulse repetitions / Half and Half Planks ™ - 3 sets of 20 seconds (each side)

Day 5 ( ) *write day*

Important: Wear your Sillo Belly Wrap ™ every night, (**start crossing in the back**).

Assessments: *(circle what applies)*
*Surge Posture: 75% or more of the day / 50% of the day / less than 25% of the day
*Core Posture: 75% or more of the day / 50% of the day / less than 25% of the day
Set Posture: 75% or more of the day / 50% of the day / less than 25% of the day
Breathe Posture: 75% or more of the day / 50% of the day / less than 25% of the day

Standing Tilts ™ - How many sets today_____.
Half and Half Planks ™ - How many sets today_____, how many seconds each set _____.

Day 6 ( ) *write day*

Assessments: *(circle what applies)*
*Surge Posture: 75% or more of the day / 50% of the day / less than 25% of the day
*Core Posture: 75% or more of the day / 50% of the day / less than 25% of the day
Set Posture: 75% or more of the day / 50% of the day / less than 25% of the day
Breathe Posture: 75% or more of the day / 50% of the day / less than 25% of the day

Standing Tilts ™ - How many sets today_____.
Half and Half Planks ™ - How many sets today_____, how many seconds each set _____.

Day 7 ( ) *write day*

Assessments: *(circle what applies)*
*Surge Posture: 75% or more of the day / 50% of the day / less than 25% of the day
*Core Posture: 75% or more of the day / 50% of the day / less than 25% of the day
Set Posture: 75% or more of the day / 50% of the day / less than 25% of the day
Breathe Posture: 75% or more of the day / 50% of the day / less than 25% of the day

Standing Tilts ™ - How many sets today_____.
Half and Half Planks ™ - How many sets today_____, how many seconds each set _____.

Ishio Method ™ Abdominal Rehab (check-off sheet)

Week 14 (/   /20   thru   /   /20   )

Write in your own personal dates.

Adding: Micro-crunches ™ and Toe Taps ™

Set: Micro-crunches ™ - 3 sets of 10-25 reps / Toe Taps ™ - 2 sets of 10 repetitions

---

Day 1 (**)** *write day*

Important: Wear your Sillo Belly Wrap ™ every night, (crossing in the front).

Assessments: *(circle what applies)*
*Surge Posture: 75% or more of the day / 50% of the day / less than 25% of the day
*Core Posture: 75% or more of the day / 50% of the day / less than 25% of the day
Set Posture: 75% or more of the day / 50% of the day / less than 25% of the day
Breathe Posture: 75% or more of the day / 50% of the day / less than 25% of the day

Micro-crunches ™ - How many sets today_____ / Toe Taps ™ - How many sets today _____.
Half and Half Planks ™ - (1 set only) How many seconds each set _____.

Day 2 (**)** *write day*

Assessments: *(circle what applies)*
*Surge Posture: 75% or more of the day / 50% of the day / less than 25% of the day
*Core Posture: 75% or more of the day / 50% of the day / less than 25% of the day
Set Posture: 75% or more of the day / 50% of the day / less than 25% of the day
Breathe Posture: 75% or more of the day / 50% of the day / less than 25% of the day

Micro-crunches ™ - How many sets today_____ / Toe Taps ™ - How many sets today _____.
Half and Half Planks ™ - (1 set only) How many seconds each set _____.

Day 3 (**)** *write day*

Assessments: *(circle what applies)*
*Surge Posture: 75% or more of the day / 50% of the day / less than 25% of the day
*Core Posture: 75% or more of the day / 50% of the day / less than 25% of the day
Set Posture: 75% or more of the day / 50% of the day / less than 25% of the day
Breathe Posture: 75% or more of the day / 50% of the day / less than 25% of the day

Micro-crunches ™ - How many sets today_____ / Toe Taps ™ - How many sets today _____.
Half and Half Planks ™ - (1 set only) How many seconds each set _____.

Day 4 (**)** *write day*

Assessments: *(circle what applies)*
*Surge Posture: 75% or more of the day / 50% of the day / less than 25% of the day
*Core Posture: 75% or more of the day / 50% of the day / less than 25% of the day
Set Posture: 75% or more of the day / 50% of the day / less than 25% of the day
Breathe Posture: 75% or more of the day / 50% of the day / less than 25% of the day

Micro-crunches ™ - How many sets today_____ / Toe Taps ™ - How many sets today _____.
Half and Half Planks ™ - (1 set only) How many seconds each set _____.

Ishio Method ™ Abdominal Rehab (check-off sheet)

Week 14 (/ /20 thru / /20)

Write in your own personal dates.

Adding: Micro-crunches ™ and Toe Taps ™

Set: Micro-crunches ™ - 3 sets of 10-25 reps / Toe Taps ™ - 2 sets of 10 repetitions

---

Day 5 (_____ **)** *write day*

> **Important:** Wear your Sillo Belly Wrap ™ every night, (crossing in the front).

Assessments: *(circle what applies)*
*Surge Posture: 75% or more of the day / 50% of the day / less than 25% of the day
*Core Posture: 75% or more of the day / 50% of the day / less than 25% of the day
Set Posture: 75% or more of the day / 50% of the day / less than 25% of the day
Breathe Posture: 75% or more of the day / 50% of the day / less than 25% of the day

Micro-crunches ™ - How many sets today_____ / Toe Taps ™ - How many sets today _____.
Half and Half Planks ™ - (1 set only) How many seconds each set _____.

Day 6 (_____ **)** *write day*

Assessments: *(circle what applies)*
*Surge Posture: 75% or more of the day / 50% of the day / less than 25% of the day
*Core Posture: 75% or more of the day / 50% of the day / less than 25% of the day
Set Posture: 75% or more of the day / 50% of the day / less than 25% of the day
Breathe Posture: 75% or more of the day / 50% of the day / less than 25% of the day

Micro-crunches ™ - How many sets today_____ / Toe Taps ™ - How many sets today _____.
Half and Half Planks ™ - (1 set only) How many seconds each set _____.

Day 7 (_____ **)** *write day*

Assessments: *(circle what applies)*
*Surge Posture: 75% or more of the day / 50% of the day / less than 25% of the day
*Core Posture: 75% or more of the day / 50% of the day / less than 25% of the day
Set Posture: 75% or more of the day / 50% of the day / less than 25% of the day
Breathe Posture: 75% or more of the day / 50% of the day / less than 25% of the day

Micro-crunches ™ - How many sets today_____ / Toe Taps ™ - How many sets today _____.
Half and Half Planks ™ - (1 set only) How many seconds each set _____.

237

Ishio Method ™ Abdominal Rehab (check-off sheet)

Week 15 (/ /20 thru / /20)

Write in your own personal dates.

Adding: Micro-crunches ™ and Toe Taps ™

Set: Micro-crunches ™ - 3 sets of 10-25 reps / Toe Taps ™ - 2 sets of 10 repetitions

Day 1 ( ) *write day*

Important: Wear your Sillo Belly Wrap ™ every night, (crossing in the front).

Assessments: *(circle what applies)*
*Surge Posture: 75% or more of the day / 50% of the day / less than 25% of the day
*Core Posture: 75% or more of the day / 50% of the day / less than 25% of the day
Set Posture: 75% or more of the day / 50% of the day / less than 25% of the day
Breathe Posture: 75% or more of the day / 50% of the day / less than 25% of the day

Micro-crunches ™ - How many sets today_____ / Toe Taps ™ - How many sets today _____.
Half and Half Planks ™ - (1 set only) How many seconds each set _____.

Day 2 ( ) *write day*

Assessments: *(circle what applies)*
*Surge Posture: 75% or more of the day / 50% of the day / less than 25% of the day
*Core Posture: 75% or more of the day / 50% of the day / less than 25% of the day
Set Posture: 75% or more of the day / 50% of the day / less than 25% of the day
Breathe Posture: 75% or more of the day / 50% of the day / less than 25% of the day

Micro-crunches ™ - How many sets today_____ / Toe Taps ™ - How many sets today _____.
Half and Half Planks ™ - (1 set only) How many seconds each set _____.

Day 3 ( ) *write day*

Assessments: *(circle what applies)*
*Surge Posture: 75% or more of the day / 50% of the day / less than 25% of the day
*Core Posture: 75% or more of the day / 50% of the day / less than 25% of the day
Set Posture: 75% or more of the day / 50% of the day / less than 25% of the day
Breathe Posture: 75% or more of the day / 50% of the day / less than 25% of the day

Micro-crunches ™ - How many sets today_____ / Toe Taps ™ - How many sets today _____.
Half and Half Planks ™ - (1 set only) How many seconds each set _____.

Day 4 ( ) *write day*

Assessments: *(circle what applies)*
*Surge Posture: 75% or more of the day / 50% of the day / less than 25% of the day
*Core Posture: 75% or more of the day / 50% of the day / less than 25% of the day
Set Posture: 75% or more of the day / 50% of the day / less than 25% of the day
Breathe Posture: 75% or more of the day / 50% of the day / less than 25% of the day

Micro-crunches ™ - How many sets today_____ / Toe Taps ™ - How many sets today _____.
Half and Half Planks ™ - (1 set only) How many seconds each set _____.

Ishio Method ™ Abdominal Rehab (check-off sheet)

Week 15 (/ /20 thru / /20)

Write in your own personal dates.

Adding: Micro-crunches ™ and Toe Taps ™

Set: Micro-crunches ™ - 3 sets of 10-25 reps / Toe Taps ™ - 2 sets of 10 repetitions

---

Day 5 ( ) *write day*

| **Important:** Wear your Sillo Belly Wrap ™ every night, (crossing in the front). |

Assessments: *(circle what applies)*
*Surge Posture: 75% or more of the day / 50% of the day / less than 25% of the day
*Core Posture: 75% or more of the day / 50% of the day / less than 25% of the day
Set Posture: 75% or more of the day / 50% of the day / less than 25% of the day
Breathe Posture: 75% or more of the day / 50% of the day / less than 25% of the day

Micro-crunches ™ - How many sets today_____ / Toe Taps ™ - How many sets today _____.
Half and Half Planks ™ - (1 set only) How many seconds each set _____.

Day 6 ( ) *write day*

Assessments: *(circle what applies)*
*Surge Posture: 75% or more of the day / 50% of the day / less than 25% of the day
*Core Posture: 75% or more of the day / 50% of the day / less than 25% of the day
Set Posture: 75% or more of the day / 50% of the day / less than 25% of the day
Breathe Posture: 75% or more of the day / 50% of the day / less than 25% of the day

Micro-crunches ™ - How many sets today_____ / Toe Taps ™ - How many sets today _____.
Half and Half Planks ™ - (1 set only) How many seconds each set _____.

Day 7 ( ) *write day*

Assessments: *(circle what applies)*
*Surge Posture: 75% or more of the day / 50% of the day / less than 25% of the day
*Core Posture: 75% or more of the day / 50% of the day / less than 25% of the day
Set Posture: 75% or more of the day / 50% of the day / less than 25% of the day
Breathe Posture: 75% or more of the day / 50% of the day / less than 25% of the day

Micro-crunches ™ - How many sets today_____ / Toe Taps ™ - How many sets today _____.
Half and Half Planks ™ - (1 set only) How many seconds each set _____.

Ishio Method ™ Abdominal Rehab (check-off sheet)

Week 16 (/   /20   thru   /   /20   )   *Write in your own personal dates.*

Adding: Micro-crunches ™ and Toe Taps ™

Set: Micro-crunches ™ - 3 sets of 10-25 reps / Toe Taps ™ - 2 sets of 10 repetitions

---

Day 1 (   ) *write day*

| **Important:** Wear your Sillo Belly Wrap ™ every night, (crossing in the front). |

Assessments: *(circle what applies)*
*Surge Posture: 75% or more of the day / 50% of the day / less than 25% of the day
*Core Posture: 75% or more of the day / 50% of the day / less than 25% of the day
Set Posture: 75% or more of the day / 50% of the day / less than 25% of the day
Breathe Posture: 75% or more of the day / 50% of the day / less than 25% of the day

Micro-crunches ™ - How many sets today_____ / Toe Taps ™ - How many sets today _____.
Half and Half Planks ™ - (1 set only) How many seconds each set _____.

Day 2 (   ) *write day*

Assessments: *(circle what applies)*
*Surge Posture: 75% or more of the day / 50% of the day / less than 25% of the day
*Core Posture: 75% or more of the day / 50% of the day / less than 25% of the day
Set Posture: 75% or more of the day / 50% of the day / less than 25% of the day
Breathe Posture: 75% or more of the day / 50% of the day / less than 25% of the day

Micro-crunches ™ - How many sets today_____ / Toe Taps ™ - How many sets today _____.
Half and Half Planks ™ - (1 set only) How many seconds each set _____.

Day 3 (   ) *write day*

Assessments: *(circle what applies)*
*Surge Posture: 75% or more of the day / 50% of the day / less than 25% of the day
*Core Posture: 75% or more of the day / 50% of the day / less than 25% of the day
Set Posture: 75% or more of the day / 50% of the day / less than 25% of the day
Breathe Posture: 75% or more of the day / 50% of the day / less than 25% of the day

Micro-crunches ™ - How many sets today_____ / Toe Taps ™ - How many sets today _____.
Half and Half Planks ™ - (1 set only) How many seconds each set _____.

Day 4 (   ) *write day*

Assessments: *(circle what applies)*
*Surge Posture: 75% or more of the day / 50% of the day / less than 25% of the day
*Core Posture: 75% or more of the day / 50% of the day / less than 25% of the day
Set Posture: 75% or more of the day / 50% of the day / less than 25% of the day
Breathe Posture: 75% or more of the day / 50% of the day / less than 25% of the day

Micro-crunches ™ - How many sets today_____ / Toe Taps ™ - How many sets today _____.
Half and Half Planks ™ - (1 set only) How many seconds each set _____.

Ishio Method ™ **Abdominal Rehab (check-off sheet)**

Week 16 (/   /20   thru   /   /20   )

Write in your own personal dates.

Adding: Micro-crunches ™ and Toe Taps ™

Set: Micro-crunches ™ - 3 sets of 10-25 reps / Toe Taps ™ - 2 sets of 10 repetitions

---

Day 5 (_____ **)** *write day*

Important: Wear your Sillo Belly Wrap ™ every night, (crossing in the front).

Assessments: *(circle what applies)*
*Surge Posture: 75% or more of the day / 50% of the day / less than 25% of the day
*Core Posture: 75% or more of the day / 50% of the day / less than 25% of the day
Set Posture: 75% or more of the day / 50% of the day / less than 25% of the day
Breathe Posture: 75% or more of the day / 50% of the day / less than 25% of the day

Micro-crunches ™ - How many sets today_____ / Toe Taps ™ - How many sets today _____.
Half and Half Planks ™ - (1 set only) How many seconds each set _____.

Day 6 (_____ **)** *write day*

Assessments: *(circle what applies)*
*Surge Posture: 75% or more of the day / 50% of the day / less than 25% of the day
*Core Posture: 75% or more of the day / 50% of the day / less than 25% of the day
Set Posture: 75% or more of the day / 50% of the day / less than 25% of the day
Breathe Posture: 75% or more of the day / 50% of the day / less than 25% of the day

Micro-crunches ™ - How many sets today_____ / Toe Taps ™ - How many sets today _____.
Half and Half Planks ™ - (1 set only) How many seconds each set _____.

Day 7 (_____ **)** *write day*

Assessments: *(circle what applies)*
*Surge Posture: 75% or more of the day / 50% of the day / less than 25% of the day
*Core Posture: 75% or more of the day / 50% of the day / less than 25% of the day
Set Posture: 75% or more of the day / 50% of the day / less than 25% of the day
Breathe Posture: 75% or more of the day / 50% of the day / less than 25% of the day

Micro-crunches ™ - How many sets today_____ / Toe Taps ™ - How many sets today _____.
Half and Half Planks ™ - (1 set only) How many seconds each set _____.

Ishio Method ™ Abdominal Rehab (check-off sheet)

Week 17 (/   /20   thru   /   /20   )   *Write in your own personal dates.*

Adding: Micro-crunches ™ and Toe Taps ™

Set: Micro-crunches ™ - 3 sets of 10-25 reps / Toe Taps ™ - 2 sets of 10 repetitions

---

Day 1 ( ) *write day*

| **Important:** Wear your Sillo Belly Wrap ™ every night, (crossing in the front). |

Assessments: *(circle what applies)*
*Surge Posture: 75% or more of the day / 50% of the day / less than 25% of the day
*Core Posture: 75% or more of the day / 50% of the day / less than 25% of the day
Set Posture: 75% or more of the day / 50% of the day / less than 25% of the day
Breathe Posture: 75% or more of the day / 50% of the day / less than 25% of the day

Micro-crunches ™ - How many sets today_____ / Toe Taps ™ - How many sets today _____.
Half and Half Planks ™ - (1 set only) How many seconds each set _____.

Day 2 ( ) *write day*

Assessments: *(circle what applies)*
*Surge Posture: 75% or more of the day / 50% of the day / less than 25% of the day
*Core Posture: 75% or more of the day / 50% of the day / less than 25% of the day
Set Posture: 75% or more of the day / 50% of the day / less than 25% of the day
Breathe Posture: 75% or more of the day / 50% of the day / less than 25% of the day

Micro-crunches ™ - How many sets today_____ / Toe Taps ™ - How many sets today _____.
Half and Half Planks ™ - (1 set only) How many seconds each set _____.

Day 3 ( ) *write day*

Assessments: *(circle what applies)*
*Surge Posture: 75% or more of the day / 50% of the day / less than 25% of the day
*Core Posture: 75% or more of the day / 50% of the day / less than 25% of the day
Set Posture: 75% or more of the day / 50% of the day / less than 25% of the day
Breathe Posture: 75% or more of the day / 50% of the day / less than 25% of the day

Micro-crunches ™ - How many sets today_____ / Toe Taps ™ - How many sets today _____.
Half and Half Planks ™ - (1 set only) How many seconds each set _____.

Day 4 ( ) *write day*

Assessments: *(circle what applies)*
*Surge Posture: 75% or more of the day / 50% of the day / less than 25% of the day
*Core Posture: 75% or more of the day / 50% of the day / less than 25% of the day
Set Posture: 75% or more of the day / 50% of the day / less than 25% of the day
Breathe Posture: 75% or more of the day / 50% of the day / less than 25% of the day

Micro-crunches ™ - How many sets today_____ / Toe Taps ™ - How many sets today _____.
Half and Half Planks ™ - (1 set only) How many seconds each set _____.

Ishio Method ™ Abdominal Rehab (check-off sheet)

Week 17 (/   /20   thru   /   /20   )   *Write in your own personal dates.*

Adding: Micro-crunches ™ and Toe Taps ™

Set: Micro-crunches ™ - 3 sets of 10-25 reps / Toe Taps ™ - 2 sets of 10 repetitions

---

Day 5 (**)** *write day*

> **Important:** Wear your Sillo Belly Wrap ™ every night, (crossing in the front).

Assessments: *(circle what applies)*
*Surge Posture: 75% or more of the day / 50% of the day / less than 25% of the day
*Core Posture: 75% or more of the day / 50% of the day / less than 25% of the day
Set Posture: 75% or more of the day / 50% of the day / less than 25% of the day
Breathe Posture: 75% or more of the day / 50% of the day / less than 25% of the day

Micro-crunches ™ - How many sets today_____ / Toe Taps ™ - How many sets today _____.
Half and Half Planks ™ - (1 set only) How many seconds each set _____.

Day 6 (**)** *write day*

Assessments: *(circle what applies)*
*Surge Posture: 75% or more of the day / 50% of the day / less than 25% of the day
*Core Posture: 75% or more of the day / 50% of the day / less than 25% of the day
Set Posture: 75% or more of the day / 50% of the day / less than 25% of the day
Breathe Posture: 75% or more of the day / 50% of the day / less than 25% of the day

Micro-crunches ™ - How many sets today_____ / Toe Taps ™ - How many sets today _____.
Half and Half Planks ™ - (1 set only) How many seconds each set _____.

Day 7 (**)** *write day*

Assessments: *(circle what applies)*
*Surge Posture: 75% or more of the day / 50% of the day / less than 25% of the day
*Core Posture: 75% or more of the day / 50% of the day / less than 25% of the day
Set Posture: 75% or more of the day / 50% of the day / less than 25% of the day
Breathe Posture: 75% or more of the day / 50% of the day / less than 25% of the day

Micro-crunches ™ - How many sets today_____ / Toe Taps ™ - How many sets today _____.
Half and Half Planks ™ - (1 set only) How many seconds each set _____.

243

My Baby Hijacked My Body,Now I Want it Back!

PostPregnancyRehab.com

Top-10 Nutrition Favorites

(Jot down the accurate calorie count next to each item)

	Breakfast	Lunch	Dinner	Snack
1.				
2.				
3.				
4.				
5.				
6.				
7.				
8.				
9.				
10.				

My Baby Hijacked My Body. Now I Want it Back!

PostPregnancyRehab.com

Top-10 Nutrition Favorites

(Jot down the accurate calorie count next to each item)

	Breakfast	Lunch	Dinner	Snack
1.	Homemade Egg & cheese sandwich 350cals	Baja Fresh 2 grilled chicken tacos, small salad 550cals	Mc Donalds cheese burger, salad, snack parfait 450cals	Yoplait Greek yogurt 110 cals
2.	T.G. waffle, 2 egg whites, orange 300 cals	Subway 6in club, baked lays 460cals	Japanese Curry 1 cup w/1 cup rice steamed peas 520cals	T.G. Vanilla protein shake w/ water 140cals
3.		Mr. Ricks slice pizza, steamed veggies 250 cals	Miyako's nabeyaki udon 475cals	Robeks - Dr Robeks 181cals
4.		2 blackened fish tacos, salad 450cals	1 1/2 Cup - chicken fried rice, plate of greens 400cals	Special K strawberry bar 90cals
5.		State fair corn dog, baked chips 350cals	Seasoned salmon, cup rice, steamed veggies 350cals	Kashi granola bar trail mix 140 cals
6.			Chicken breast (no skin), 1 1/2 cups mashed potatoes, broccoli 400cals	Sunchips multi grain snacks 140cals
7.				Yogurt pretzels trails mix 150cals
8.				Japanese vegetable chips pack 130cals
9.				Yogurt raisins 150cals
10.				carrots and ranch snack pack X 2 140cals

My Baby Hijacked My Body, Now I Want it Back!

PostPregnancyRehab.com

Weekly Training Plan

Monday: Training

Tuesday: Training

Wednesday: Training

Thursday: Training

Friday: Training

Saturday: Training

Sunday: Training

Notes:

My Baby Hijacked My Body, Now I Want it Back!

PostPregnancyRehab.com

Weekly Training Plan

Monday: Training
9am – Cardio Kick box class
Stretch

Tuesday: Training
8:30am – Jog 30min (baby jogger)
Stretch

Wednesday: Training
8:30am – Jog 20min
Weights 30min (all major muscle groups)
Stretch

Thursday: Training
8am – Park Boot Camp

Friday: Training
8:30am – Jog 20min
Weights 30min (all major muscle groups)
Stretch

Saturday: Training
Scheduled Day-off

Sunday: Training
Scheduled Day-off

Notes:

My Baby Hijacked My Body, Now I Want it Back!

PostPregnancyRehab.com

Lifestyle Log

Week:

(Fill this part out AFTER the week has been completed)

Nutrition Score (circle one)

Just right   Not quite   Way off

Training Score (how many days you trained, marked over, how many days you plan to train – example 5/5)

Notes to self

Date/Day:

Wake-up:

Time/What:

Time/What:

Time/What:

Time/What:

Time/What:

Time/What:

Time/What:

Bedtime:

My Baby Hijacked My Body, Now I Want it Back!
PostPregnancyRehab.com

Lifestyle Log
(day two and three)

Date/Day:

Wake-up:

Time/What:

Time/What:

Time/What:

Time/What:

Time/What:

Time/What:

Time/What:

Bedtime:

Date/Day:

Wake-up:

Time/What:

Time/What:

Time/What:

Time/What:

Time/What:

Time/What:

Time/What:

Bedtime:

My Baby Hijacked My Body, Now I Want it Back!
PostPregnancyRehab.com

Lifestyle Log
(day four and five)

Date/Day:

Wake-up:

Time/What:

Time/What:

Time/What:

Time/What:

Time/What:

Time/What:

Time/What:

Bedtime:

Date/Day:

Wake-up:

Time/What:

Time/What:

Time/What:

Time/What:

Time/What:

Time/What:

Time/What:

Bedtime:

Lifestyle Log
(day six and seven)

Date/Day:

Wake-up:

Time/What:

Time/What:

Time/What:

Time/What:

Time/What:

Time/What:

Time/What:

Bedtime:

Date/Day:

Wake-up:

Time/What:

Time/What:

Time/What:

Time/What:

Time/What:

Time/What:

Time/What:

Bedtime:

My Baby Hijacked My Body, Now I Want it Back!
PostPregnancyRehab.com

Lifestyle Log

Week: *April 5th – 11th, 2010*

(Fill this part out AFTER the week has been completed)

Nutrition Score (circle one)   *because of the weekends only*

Just right (**Not quite**) **Way off**

Training Score (how many days you trained, marked over, how many days you plan to train – example 5/5)   *4/5 – ditched my scheduled weekend work-out*

Notes to self

Mon – Fri I do well, but weekends are tough with my eating and working out. I will pre-plan most of my weekend meals and start doing my "scheduled day-offs" on the weekends too. I need to make it work because what I was doing wasn't and I deserve it.

Date/Day: *4/5/10 – Mon*

Total 1283 cals

Wake-up: *6:45 am*

Time/What: *7:45am – 1 cup oatmeal and banana (200 cal)*

Time/What: *8:30am – Park Bootcamp 1 hour (pushed myself more than usual)*

Time/What: *10am – small handfull nuts and small plum (110 cal)*

Time/What: *11:45am – turkey sandwich w/lettuce, sm cookie (350 cal)*

Time/What: *2:45pm – string cheese, 2 big strawberry's (103 cal)*

Time/What: *6:46pm – Chicken breast, 1 2 hawaiian bread, steamed*

Time/What: *broccoli with little butter/pepper/salt*

small piece cake (520cal)

Bedtime: *10:45pm*

My Baby Hijacked My Body, Now I Want it Back!
PostPregnancyRehab.com

Training Check-off

Week: / / - / /

Mon: ☐

Tue: ☐

Wed: ☐

Thu: ☐

Fri: ☐

Sat: ☐

Sun: ☐

Week: / / - / /

Mon: ☐

Tue: ☐

Wed: ☐

Thu: ☐

Fri: ☐

Sat: ☐

Sun: ☐

Week: / / - / /

Mon: ☐

Tue: ☐

Wed: ☐

Thu: ☐

Fri: ☐

Sat: ☐

Sun: ☐

Week: / / - / /

Mon: ☐

Tue: ☐

Wed: ☐

Thu: ☐

Fri: ☐

Sat: ☐

Sun: ☐

My Baby Hijacked My Body, Now I Want it Back!

PostPregnancyRehab.com

Training Check-off

Week: 0 / 00 / 00 - 0 / 00 / 0   **Week:** 0 / 00 / 00 - 0 / 00 / 0

Mon: [X] Scheduled Day Off   **Mon:** [X] Scheduled Day Off

                                                                  Didn't do :-(

Tue: [X] Jog (15 minutes)   **Tue:** [ ] Jog (15 minutes)
         Weights at gym (30 minutes)   Weights at gym (30 minutes)

Wed: [X] Class at Kens Martial Arts   **Wed:** [X] Class at Kens Martial Arts
         "Cardio Kick boxing" (60 min)   "Cardio Kick boxing" (60 min)

Thu: [X] Jog (15 minutes)   **Thu:** [X] Jog (15 minutes)
         Weights at gym (30 minutes)   Weights at gym (30 minutes)

Fri: [X] Jog / Walk Intervals   **Fri:** [X] Jog / Walk Intervals
         (10min warmup, 7 X 1 min jogs   (10min warmup, 7 X 1 min jogs
         alt 7 X min walk, 5min cooldown)   alt 7 X min walk, 5min cooldown

Sat: [X] Scheduled Day Off   **Sat:** [X] Scheduled Day Off

     30min jog instead - kids at party
Sun: [X] ~~Play tag with kids (30-45 min)~~   **Sun:** [X] Play tag with kids (30-45 min)

Week: / / - / /   **Week:** / / - / /

Mon: [ ] Scheduled Day Off   **Mon:** [ ] Scheduled Day Off

Tue: [ ] Jog (15 minutes)   **Tue:** [ ] Jog (15 minutes)
         Weights at gym (30 minutes)   Weights at gym (30 minutes)

Wed: [ ] Class at Kens Martial Arts   **Wed:** [ ] Class at Kens Martial Arts
         "Cardio Kick boxing" (60 min)   "Cardio Kick boxing" (60 min)

Thu: [ ] Jog (15 minutes)   **Thu:** [ ] Jog (15 minutes)
         Weights at gym (30 minutes)   Weights at gym (30 minutes)

Fri: [ ] Jog / Walk Intervals   **Fri:** [ ] Jog / Walk Intervals
         (10min warmup, 7 X 1 min jogs   (10min warmup, 7 X 1 min jogs
         alt 7 X min walk, 5min cooldown)   alt 7 X min walk, 5min cooldown

Sat: [ ] Scheduled Day Off   **Sat:** [ ] Scheduled Day Off

Sun: [ ] Play tag with kids (30-45 min)   **Sun:** [ ] Play tag with kids (30-45 min)

REFERENCES

Norton P. Pelvic floor disorders: the role of fascia and ligaments. 1993. Clinical Obstetrics and Gynecology 36;926

Snooks S, Swash M, Mathers S, Henry M. 1990. Effect of vaginal delivery on the pelvic floor: a 5-year follow-up. British Journal of Surgery 77;1358

Mathias et al. 1996 (study of how many women suffer from chronic pelvic pain).
Arnold H. Kegel, M.D., F.A.C.S.Assistant Professor of GynecologyUniversity of Southern California School of Medicine1948.

Allen R, Hosker G, Smith A, Warrell D. Pelvic floor damage and childbirth: a neurophysiologic study. 1990 British Journal of Obstetrics and Gynecology 97;770

Handa V, Harris T, Ostergard D. 1996. Protecting the pelvic floor: Obstetric management to prevent incontinence and pelvic organ prolapse. Obstetrics and Gynecology 88;470

Meyer S, Hohlfeld P, Achtari C, De Grandi P. 2001. Pelvic floor education after vagianl delivery. Obstetrics and Gynecology 97;673

Brown, JE, JNE 24:21-5, 1992 (components of weight gain). Center for population Research 1999 (pelvis floor top 3 dysfunction).

Christina Christie PT, Rich Colosi DPT, Paving the way for a healthy pelvic floor; page 3 (PCNS Anatomy) – page 4 (Muscular Support of the PCNS), May 2009.

U.S. National Library of Medicine. Informed Health Online. Ncbi.nlm.nih.gov/pubmedhealth/PMH0005004. Fact sheet: Weight gain in pregnancy. June 2009

The American College of Obstetricians and Gynecologists, FAQ0119 Pregnancy - Exercise During Pregnancy Frequently Asked Questions, August 2011

The American College of Obstetricians and Gynecologists, Exercise During Pregnancy and the Postpartum Period, Number 267 Committee Opinion, January 2002.
Rao AV, Rao LG. Carotenoids and human health. Pharmacol Res. 2007 Mar;55(3):207-16. Epub 2007 Jan 25

Evans JA, Johnson EJ. The role of phytonutrients in skin health. Nutrients. 2010 Aug;2(8):903-28. Epub 2010 Aug 24

Shi J, Le Maguer M. Lycopene in tomatoes: chemical and physical properties affected by food processing. Crit Rev Food Sci Nutr. 2000 Jan;40(1):1-42

Alda LM, Gogoasa I, Bordean DM, et al. Lycopene content of tomatoes and tomato products. Journal of Agroalimentary Processes and Technologies. 2009;15(4):540-542

Shi J, Qu Q, Kakuda Y, Yeung D, Jiang Y. Stability and synergistic effect of antioxidative properties of lycopene and other active components. Critical Reviews in Food Science and Nutrition. 2004;44:559—73

Chang MW. Disorders of hyperpigmentation. In: Bolognia JL, Jorizzo JL, Rapini RP, editors. Dermatology. 2nd ed. Elsevier Mosby; 2009. pp. 333–389

Taylor SC, Grimes PE, Lim J, et al. Postinflammatory Hyperpigmentation. J Cutan Med Surg. 2009;13:183–191

Grimes PE. Managment of hyperpigmentation in darker racial ethnic groups. Semin Cutan Med Surg. 2009;28:77–85

Lacz NL, Vafaie J, Kihiczac NI, et al. Postinflammatory hyperpigmentation: a common but troubling condition. Int J Dermatol. 2004;4:362–365

Palumbo A, d'Ischia M, Misuraca G, et al. Mechanism of inhibition of melanogenesis by hydroquinone. Biochim Biophys Acta. 1991;1073:85–90

Jimbow K, Minamitsuji Y. Topical therapies for melasma and disorders of hyperpigmentation. Dermatol Ther. 2001;14:35–45

Draelos ZD. Skin lightening preparations and the hydroquinone controversy. Dermatol Ther. 2007;20:308–313

Leu D, Yoo SS. Epidermal and color improvment in ethnic skin: microdermabrasion and superficial peels. In: Alam M, Bhatia AC, Kundu RV, Yoo SS, Chan HH, editors. Cosmetic Dermatology for Skin of Color. McGraw Hill; New York, NY: 2009. pp. 29–33

Song JY, Kang HA, Kim MY, et al. Damage and recovery of skin barrier function after glycolic acid chemical peeling and crystal microdermabrasion. Dermatol Surg. 2004;30:390–394

http://laserandveinclinic.com, Titan Laser. 2012.

http://www.fraxel.comconsumer/fraxel-difference/fraxel-science, Fraxel Laser. 2012.

Ahn HH, Kim IH. Whitening effect of salicyclic acid peels in Asian patients. Dermatol Surg. 2006;32:372–375

Ejaz A, Raza N, Iftikhar N, et al. Comparison of 30% salicylic acid with Jessner's solution for superficial chemical peeling in epidermal melasma. J Coll Physicians Surg Pak. 2008;18:205–208

American Academy of Dermatology. http://www.aad.org, melasma, signs and symptoms, who gets and causes, diagnosis, treatment, and outcome. 2012

Katz TM, Goldberg LH, Firoz BF, et al. Fractional photothermolysis for the treatment of postinflammatory hyperpigmentation. Dermatol Surg. 2009;35:1844–1848

Hesse S, Barthel H, Murai T, et al. Is correction for age necessary in neuroimaging studies of the central serotonin transporter? Eur J Nucl Med Mol Imaging. 2003 Mar;30(3):427-30

Kuikka JT, Tammela L, Bergstrom KA, et al. Effects of ageing on serotonin transporters in healthy females. Eur J Nucl Med. 2001 Jul;28(7):911-3

Porter RJ, Mulder RT, Joyce PR, Miller AL, Kennedy M. Tryptophan hydroxylase gene (TPH1) and peripheral tryptophan levels in depression. J Affect Disord. 2008 Jan 4

Booij L, Van der Does AJ, Haffmans PM, Riedel WJ, Fekkes D, Blom MJ. The effects of high-dose and low-dose tryptophan depletion on mood and cognitive functions of remitted depressed patients. J Psychopharmacol. 2005 May;19(3):267-75

Crawford S, Venzon C, Top 10 Foods High in Omega-3. 2010 Jun;15.

Post Partum Support International. Post Partum Psychosis. www.postpratum.net. Accessed 2010

Almeida-Montes LG, Valles-Sanchez V, Moreno-Aguilar J, et al. Relation of serum cholesterol, lipid, serotonin and tryptophan levels to severity of depression and to suicide attempts. J Psychiatry Neurosci. 2000 Sep;25(4):371-7

Herrington RN, Bruce A, Johnstone EC, Lader MH. Comparative trial of L-tryptophan and amitriptyline in depressive illness. Psychol Med. 1976 Nov;6(4):673-8

Kaye WH, Gendall KA, Fernstrom MH, et al. Effects of acute tryptophan depletion on mood in bulimia nervosa. Biol Psychiatry. 2000 Jan 15;47(2):151-7

Caruso C, Lio D, Cavallone L, Franceschi C. Aging, longevity, inflammation, and cancer. Ann NY Acad Sci. 2004 Dec;1028:1-13

Kiecolt-Glaser JK, Belury MA, Porter K, et al. Depressive symptoms, omega-6:omega-3 fatty acids, and inflammation in older adults. Psychosom Med. 2007 Apr;69(3):217-24

Wu D, Han SN, Meydani M, Meydani SN. Effect of concomitant consumption of fish oil and vitamin E on production of inflammatory cytokines in healthy elderly humans. Ann NY Acad Sci. 2004 Dec;1031:422-4

Katiyar SK. Skin photoprotection by green tea: antioxidant and immunomodulatory effects. Curr Drug Targets Immune Endocr Metabol Disord. 2003 Sep;3(3):234-42

Tipoe GL, Leung TM, Hung MW, Fung ML. Green tea polyphenols as an anti-oxidant and anti-inflammatory agent for cardiovascular protection. Cardiovasc Hematol Disord Drug Targets. 2007 Jun;7(2):135-44

Rothman D, DeLuca P, Zurier RB. Botanical lipids: effects on inflammation, immune responses, and rheumatoid arthritis. Semin Arthritis Rheum. 1995 Oct;25(2):87-96

O'Leary KA, de Pascual-Tereasa S, Needs PW, et al. Effect of flavonoids and vitamin E on cyclooxygenase-2 (COX-2) transcription. Mutat Res. 2004 Jul 13;551(1-2):245-54

Murakami A, Nakamura Y, Ohto Y, et al. Suppressive effects of citrus fruits on free radical generation and nobiletin, an anti-inflammatory polymethoxyflavonoid. Biofactors. 2000;12(1-4):187-92

Oxenkrug GF. Genetic and Hormonal Regulation of Tryptophan Kynurenine Metabolism: Implications for Vascular Cognitive Impairment, Major Depressive Disorder, and Aging. Ann NY Acad Sci. 2007 Dec;1122:35-49

Widner B, Laich A, Sperner-Unterweger B, Ledochowski M, Fuchs D. Neopterin production, tryptophan degradation, and mental depression—what is the link? Brain Behav Immun. 2002 Oct;16(5):590-5

Lin PY, Su KP. A meta-analytic review of double-blind, placebo-controlled trials of antidepressant efficacy of omega-3 fatty acids. J Clin Psychiatry. 2007 Jul;68(7):1056-61

Wirleitner B, Neurauter G, Schrocksnadel K, Frick B, Fuchs D. Interferon-gamma-induce conversion of tryptophan: immunologic and neuropsychiatric aspects. Curr Med Chem. 2003 Aug;10(16):1581-91

Hartmann E. Effects of L-tryptophan on sleepiness and on sleep. J Psychiatr Res. 1982;17(2):107-13.

Schneider-Helmert D, Spinweber CL. Evaluation of L-tryptophan for treatment of insomnia: a review. Psychopharmacology (Berl). 1986;89(1):1-7

Korner E, Bertha G, Flooh E, et al. Sleep-inducing effect of L-tryptophane. Eur Neurol. 1986;25(Suppl 2):75-81

Demisch K, Bauer J, Georgi K, Demisch L. Treatment of severe chronic insomnia with L-tryptophan: results of a double-blind cross-over study. Pharmacopsychiatry. 1987 Nov;20(6):242-4

Smith KA, Williams C, Cowen PJ. Impaired regulation of brain serotonin function during dieting in women recovered from depression. Br J Psychiatry. 2000 Jan;176:72-5

Guilarte TR, Wagner HN Jr. Increased concentrations of 3-hydroxykynurenine in vitamin B6 deficient neonatal rat brain. J Neurochem. 1987 Dec;49(6):1918-26

Bell C, Abrams J, Nutt D. Tryptophan depletion and its implications for psychiatry. Br J Psychiatry 2001 May;178:399-405. 2001. PMID:15990

Groff JL, Gropper SS, Hunt SM. Advanced Nutrition and Human Metabolism. West Publishing Company, New York, 1995. 1995

Martinez A, Knappskog PM, Haavik J. A structural approach into human tryptophan hydroxylase and its implications for the regulation of serotonin biosynthesis. Curr Med Chem 2001 Jul;8(9):1077-91. 2001. PMID:15980

Moore P, Landolt HP, Seifritz E, et al. Clinical and physiological consequences of rapid tryptophan depletion. Neuropsychopharmacology 2000 Dec;23(6):601-22. 2000. PMID:16020

Van der Does AJ. The effects of tryptophan depletion on mood and psychiatric symptoms. J Affect Disord 2001 May;64(2-3):107-19. 2001. PMID:16000
Urinary Neurotransmitter Testing: Problems and Alternatives, by Julia Ross, MA, MFT for the Townsend Letter (10/06)

Textbook of Dermatology. Ed Rook A, Wilkinson DS, Ebling FJB, Champion RH, Burton JL. Fourth edition. Blackwell Scientific Publications

http://www.mypyramid.gov.

health.gov/dietaryguidelines/dga2010/DietaryGuidelines2010.pdf

Department of Biology of Physical Activity. Leucine supplementation and intensive training. University of Jyväskylä, Finland. 1999 Jun;27(6):347-58

European Journal of Pharmaceutics and Biopharmaceutics. Volume 73, Pages 187 – 194, doi: 10.1016/j.ejpb.2009.04.017

Stahl, Schwarz, Sundquist, A.R. and Sies (1992) Cis-transisomers of lycopene and B-carotene in human serum and tissues, Arch. Biochem. Biophys. 294: 173-177

A.V. Rao, L.G. Rao. Carotenoids and human health. Pharmacological Research 55 (2007) 207–216

Office of Dietary Health, National Institutes of Health – Government. Dietary Supplement Fact Sheet: Valerian. 2013; 1-1

Morin CM, et al. Insomnia: Nature, diagnosis, and treatment. In: Chokroverty S, et al. Handbook of Clinical Neurology. 3rd ed. Philadelphia, Pa.: Elsevier; 2011:723

Krystal AD. Pharmacologic treatment: Other medications. In: Kryger MH, et al. Principles and Practice of Sleep Medicine. 5th ed. St. Louis, Mo.: Elsevier Saunders; 2011:916

Akhondzadeh S, Naghavi HR, Shayeganpour A, et al. Passionflower in the treatment of generalized anxiety: a pilot double-blind randomized controlled trial with oxazepam. J Clin Pharm Ther 2001;26:363-7

Bourin M, Bougerol T, Guitton B, Broutin E. A combination of plant extracts in the treatment of outpatients with adjustment disorder with anxious mood: controlled study vs placebo. Fundam Clin Pharmacol 1997;11:127-32

William W. Deardorff, PhD, ABPP. Non-Benzodiazepine Sleep Aides. www.spine-health.com. 2006; 1-4

Valerian. Natural Medicines Comprehensive Database. www.naturaldatabase.com. Accessed Sept. 16, 2011

Melatonin. Natural Medicines Comprehensive Database. www.naturaldatabase.com. Accessed Sept. 16, 2011

Office of Dietary Health, National Institutes of Health – Government. Dietary Supplement Fact Sheet: Calcium. 2013; 1-1

Office of Dietary Health, National Institutes of Health – Government. Dietary Supplement Fact Sheet: Magnesium. 2013; 1-1

Simon N. Young Are SAMe and 5-HTP safe and effective treatments for depression J Psychiatry Neurosci. 2003 November; 28(6): 471. PMCID: PMC257800

U.S. Department of Health and Services, S-Adenosyl-L-Methionine (SAMe) for Depression, Osteoarthritis, and Liver Disease, AHRQ Publication 2002; # 02-E033

U.S. Department of Health and Services, Omega-3 Fatty Acids, Effects on Mental Health, AHRQ Publication 2005; University of Ottawa Evidence-based Practice Center # 290-02-0021; Evidence Report/Technology Assessment No. 116

U.S. Department of Health and Services, Omega-3 Fatty Acids, Effects on Child and Maternal Health, AHRQ Publication 2005; Evidence Report/Technology Assessment: Number 118

U.S. Department of Health and Services, Melatonin, Treatment of Sleep Disorders, AHRQ Publication 2004; Evidence Report/Technology Assessment: Number 108

U.S. Department of Health and Services, Physical Activity, General Population and Cancer Patients and Survivors, AHRQ Publication 2004; University of Minnesota Evidence-based Practice Center, under Contract No. 290-02-0009; Evidence Report/Technology Assessment No. 10

U.S. Department of Health and Services, Treatment of Depression—Newer Pharmacotherapies, AHRQ Publication 1999; University of Texas Health Science Center at San Antonio under contract No. 290-97-0012

U.S. Department of Health and Services, *Perinatal Depression: Prevalence, Screening Accuracy, and Screening Outcomes*, AHRQ Publication 2005; RTI-University of North Carolina Evidence-based Practice Center under Contract No. 290-02-0016; Evidence Report/Technology Assessment No. 119

Seaward BL. Managing Stress: Principles and Strategies for Health and Well-Being. 6th ed. Sudbury, Mass.: Jones & Bartlett Publishers; 2009:512

Lehrer PM, et al. Principles and Practice of Stress Management. 3rd ed. New York, N.Y.: Guilford Press; 2007:333

Strohle A. Physical activity, exercise, depression and anxiety disorders. Journal of Neural Transmission. 2009;116:777

Barbour K, et al. Exercise as a treatment for depression and other psychiatric disorders. Journal of Cardiopulmonary Rehabilitation and Prevention. 2007;27:359

Donna E. Stewart, MD, FRCPC E. Robertson, M.Phil, PhD Cindy-Lee Dennis, RN, PhD Sherry L. Grace, MA, PhD Tamara Wallington, MA, MD, FRCPC. Postpartum depression: literature review of risk factors and interventions. University Health Network Women's Health Program 2003; 16-27, 60-61

C. NEILL EPPERSON, M.D. Postpartum Major Depression: Detection and Treatment. Yale University School of Medicine, New Haven, Connecticut
Am Fam Physician. 1999 Apr 15;59(8):2247-2254

Post Partum Support International. Post Partum Psychosis. www.postpratum.net. Accessed 2010

Post Partum Support International. Depression During Pregnancy and Postpartum. www.postpratum.net. Accessed 2010

Bill Gottlieb, Alternative Cures: The Most Effective Natural Home Remedies for 160 Health Problems. June 2002

Doreen Virtue, Ph.D., Constant Craving: What Your Food Cravings Mean and How to Overcome Them. September 2011

APC / Elite Books, Healing Our Planet, Healing Our Selves: The Power of change Within to Change the World. 2004

Phyllis A. Balch, CNC, Prescription for Nutritional Healing, 4th Edition: A Practical A-to-Z Reference to Drug-Free Remedies Using Vitamins, Minerals, Herbs & Food Supplements

Michael T. Murray, N.D., Joseph E. Pizzorno, N.D., Encyclopedia of Natural Medicine, Revised Second Edition

Phyllis A. Balch, CNC, Prescription for Nutritional Healing, 4th Edition: A Practical A-to-Z Reference to Drug-Free Remedies Using Vitamins, Minerals, Herbs & Food Supplements

Harris Benedict Equation / BMR calculation

Johnstone, A.M. et al. (2005). Factors influencing variation in basal metabolic rate include fat-free mass, fat mass, age and circulating thyroxine, but not sex, circulating leptin or triiodothyronine. *American Journal of Clinical Nutrition*, 82, 5, 941–948

Van Dale, D., Saris, W.H., ten Hoor, F. (1990). Weight maintenance and resting metabolic rate 18–40 months after a diet/exercise treatment. *International Journal of Obesity*, 14, 4, 347–359

About The Author:

Michelle Ishio, also known as *"Lady Action"*, grew up in Kobe, Japan, before moving to San Diego, California, during her 4th grade school year. She moved to Los Angeles, California, after being recruited to run collegiate track and field and cross-country. After receiving her degree 4-years later, she decided to stay in Los Angeles to take advantage of the multitude of opportunities that America's second largest city offers.

Michelle's expertise comes from 2 decades as an American Council on Exercise certified personal fitness trainer; certified by the Gray Institute in "Applied Functional Science"; and a Longevity & Wellness Specialist. This includes 2 decades of formal continuing education, (with specialties in women's health, and wellness). Michelle is also experienced as an elite level competitive athlete in multiple sports, (gaining in-depth understanding of injury prevention, injury management, and prompt injury rehabilitation). As well, Michelle successfully went through the post-pregnancy rehab process 3 times herself, (including postpartum depression).

Not only is Michelle creator of the Ishio Method - Post-Pregnancy Abdominal and Pelvic Floor Rehab Principles and Protocols TM, she is also the CEO/Founder of PostPregnancyRehab.com. Michelle also created the Baby Belly Jelly TM, (an anti-inflammatory and moisturizing emollient for growing and postpartum bellies), and created the Sillo Belly Wrap TM, (with a specific design to target closing the postpartum abdominal separation).

Athletically speaking, Michelle was a professional kick boxer, (former world-championed full-contact fighter). She is black belt ranked in Kung Fu & Karate. Michelle has also appeared on the TV shows American Ninja Warrior, & American Gladiators. An on-going practicing martial artist, Michelle has added obstacle course training to her regimen, and now stronger than ever.

Michelle was also an 11-year member of Track West, (an elite level track & field club), where she had her most growth as a competitive runner, and trained and competed with some of the top U.S. runners. Her specialty events are the 800 meters, 1500 meters, (and previously included the 3000 meter steeplechase). Michelle still competes in racing competitions monthly.

Through all of her experiences and accomplishments in the sports & fitness industry, it lead her to many opportunities as a professional sports & fitness model for top companies in the industry; with the ads, commercials, and magazines, having been published/aired nationally and internationally, (Nike, Muscle and Fitness Hers magazine, Kung-fu magazine, etc.)

One of the things Michelle notes that she is proud of from her travels within the fitness industry is that, with friendly encouragement/convincing, many of her clients has competed in Martial Arts, 5K, Track, Marathon, or Triathlon competitions; she is one of their biggest fans.

Believing that everyone needs to have a creative outlet of some sort, Michelle satisfies her thirst for creativity in a variety of ways, but her main outlet is doing computer graphic and web design for her businesses, (from designing all the logos, making web and print marketing materials, to even designing the covers of her books).

Michelle believes that by authentically committing yourself to your purposes and goals, you can develop impervious optimism, which will allow unlimited creativity, achievements, and peace/happiness for your heart/mind/spirit.

262

Made in the USA
Lexington, KY
17 March 2019